# SUPERGUIDES

# HERBS
## AND MEDICINAL PLANTS

## MADGE HOOPER

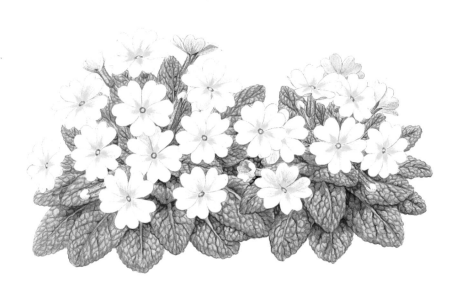

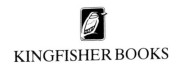

KINGFISHER BOOKS

Kingfisher Books, Grisewood & Dempsey Ltd,
Elsley House, 24–30 Great Titchfield Street
London W1P 7AD

This edition published in 1989 by Kingfisher Books.
Material in this book was first published in 1984
in the Kingfisher Guide series.

British Library Cataloguing in Publication Data
Hooper, Madge
    Herbs and medicinal plants.
    1. Herbs 2. Medicinal plants
    I. Title II. Series
    641-3'57

ISBN 0-86272-484-8

Illustrated by Sarah De Ath and George Thompson

Edited by Janice Lacock
Designed by Millions Design
Printed in Hong Kong

# CONTENTS

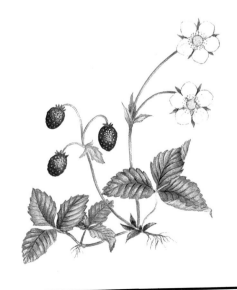

# INTRODUCTION

Over thousands of years, herbs have been used as food, or to make food more palatable, as important drugs and simple medicinal remedies, and as sweet-smelling plants which give pleasure. The earliest cave-dwellers discovered that eating certain plants improved their diet and health. They also found that plants could provide fibre for clothing and dyes to colour body and fabric, and could be used to make signs, drawings and paintings. Most important of all, perhaps, certain herbs could be used to relieve and sometimes cure the ailments which were an inevitable part of hard and dangerous lives. Fear, superstition and magic were often entangled with herbal treatment in the past but modern research, which can analyse the plants into their constituents, has finally established the sound scientific basis of much herbal medicine.

## HARVESTING AND DRYING HERBS

Even a small herb garden, once it is established, can produce more growth during the summer than will be needed for immediate use, so the surplus can be dried or frozen. In drying, herbs should lose nothing but their moisture, retaining both colour and fragrance. Whether they are to be used for cooking, herb teas or in pot pourri, the principles of drying are the same. When the herb is coming into flower, the oil content of the plant and the source of flavour and scent held in the stem and leaves are at their highest, so when possible this is the best time to harvest them.

To dry herbs well they need a steady circulation of heat, and light must be excluded to preserve their colour. Trying to dry them by hanging them in bunches in an airy place will usually lead to disappointment. The inside of a bunch does not dry as quickly as the outside, and the airy place may be dry during the day and moist at night. At home, the airing cupboard with its slatted shelves over the hot water cylinder makes an ideal place to dry small quantities of herbs and flowers. Some loosely woven material or netting can be spread over the shelves, the herbs can be put in baskets or, best of all, in one or two wooden or metal framed sieves, diameter 14in or 18in with mesh $\frac{1}{4}$in and $\frac{1}{8}$in.

The herbs should be cut on a dry morning when the dew is gone, and before the sun gets too hot. Always cut the plants a few centimetres above ground level to avoid any mud-splashed leaves, and discard those which are discoloured. Fresh herbs should be handled as little as possible to avoid bruising them – once they have lost their colour they cannot regain it. Put the herbs into the sieves and then the sieves into the airing cupboard. Turn the herbs over carefully the following day and each day after that till they are crisp and the stems snap when bent; 3–5 days is usually long enough for them to dry, but small-leaved herbs like thyme dry more quickly than those with bigger, fleshier leaves.

## PREPARING DRIED HERBS

When all the material is completely dry, take the sieve from the airing cupboard and put some sheets of clean paper on a table. Wearing a glove to avoid getting splinters in the palm, rub the herbs through the mesh with a firm circular movement of the flat hand so that the stalks lie horizontally on top of the sieve and the crushed herb falls through. Throw away the big stalks, tip the rubbed herbs back into the sieve and repeat the process.

If the herb is to be used as an infusion, two rubs through the $\frac{1}{4}$in. mesh will be sufficient to get rid of most of the stalks. Herbs to be used in cooking should be rubbed through the $\frac{1}{8}$in. mesh, reducing the size of the rubbed herb and eliminating all stalks. A close mesh metal, hair or nylon sieve is useful to shake the rubbed herbs in: any dust will fall through, leaving the herbs clean and ready for storing.

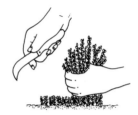

1. Cut herbs a little above ground level to avoid leaves mud-splashed from rain.

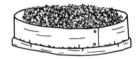

2. Fill the sieve with lightly packed cut herbs.

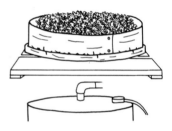

3. Place sieve in a warm airing cupboard or other warm, darkish place, to dry.

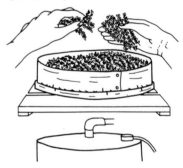

4. Lightly turn herbs daily to ensure even drying. Do not bruise leaves when handling them.

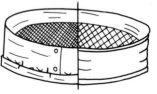

Wooden sieve      Metal sieve
$\frac{1}{8}$in. (0.3cm) mesh   $\frac{1}{4}$in. (0.6cm) mesh

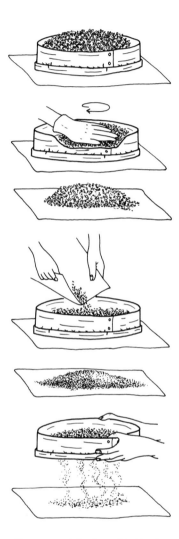

*To extract stalks from dried herbs, rub the herbs through a sieve.*

## STORING HERBS

It is as important to store herbs out of direct light as it is to dry them in the dark. They should be kept in glass jars with well-fitting screw on lids lined with greaseproof paper or foil. For large quantities, use strong brown paper bags enclosed in plastic bags and carefully sealed with twist ties. With the exception of parsley, which always fades after a few months, herbs stored in these conditions should last until the following summer's crops can replace them.

Herbs for freezing should be carefully selected, washed and shaken free of excess moisture. They can then be packed in the small amounts usually needed, and stored together in clearly labelled bags or boxes. Parsley, thyme, sage, rosemary and bay usually survive the winter and can be picked fresh from the garden, but well dried herbs make welcome presents for friends without gardens. Bay leaves should be picked when they are quite dry, and only the stiff, mature leaves used. If they are loosely wrapped, ten at a time, in greaseproof paper or foil, and then enclosed in sealed brown paper bags, they will stay a good green colour for some time. Dried bay leaves will lose their colour and break up. The subtle use of herbs in cooking is an old skill which is being relearned in this country, and one which offers endless opportunities to explore the scope of a wide variety of herbs. The best cooks are not always the ones who use the same recipes every time, but those who experiment with flair.

## MAKING POT POURRI

The flowers and scented herbs used in pot pourri dry excellently in the airing cupboard. Rose petals, the most important ingredient, should be taken from fully open roses the day before they would have dropped (this soon becomes easy to judge). Cornflowers, marigolds and delphiniums have no scent but they add good colour to the mixture. Some flowers, particularly those which grow from spring bulbs, do not hold their colour well, but it is best to experiment at first with what is in your garden. Lavender, rosemary, scented mints, clove carnations, lemon verbena, bergamot and other scented flowers, blended with rose petals, will make a delightful pot pourri. It is tempting to try out the recipes in old herb books, but some of the gums, oils and spices they mention are expensive and very difficult to obtain. Orris powder 'fixes' or holds the perfumes of the other ingredients; and peel of oranges, lemons, tangerines or satsumas, dried in a cool oven until crisp, then put through a grinder and added to the mixture, will also act as a fixing agent.

Pot pourri should not have a heavy scent, but a light elusive perfume needing just a stir of the hand to refresh it. It is pleasant to have it in open bowls in a room, but it will keep its colour and fragrance longer if it can be stored in a covered jar.

## ABOUT THIS BOOK

The herbs described in this book grow wild or can be cultivated in northern Europe, and many are commonly known in North America, Australasia and other parts of the world. Even between northern and southern Britain there are variations in weather patterns, so a general guide to the seasons in which plants flower is given rather than specific months. Soil and climatic conditions affect the ultimate size to which plants grow so the heights should be taken as an approximate guide.

> **WARNING**
> Some herbs look similar to other poisonous plants at certain times of the year, so it is vital to identify any plant correctly before using it as an infusion or foodstuff. If in doubt, do not use.
> In addition, herbs which are beneficial in small doses may cause unpleasant reactions if excessive amounts are taken. Do not exceed the stated amounts.

## Family Boraginaceae

### ALKANET
(Evergreen Alkanet)
*Pentaglottis sempervirens*

A persistent hardy perennial (to 26in) which remains in leaf during the winter. Its root is thick, branching and dark-skinned. The pointed, ovate leaves are up to 12in long and 6in wide, with a noticeable network of veins. Both the stalk and the leaves are hairy. The rich blue flowers, like large forget-me-nots, are arranged on one side of short spikes and bloom from late spring to autumn. The fresh green foliage is welcome in winter, but the plant spreads rapidly and is best in informal settings.

**Cultivation:** plant in spring or autumn. Will tolerate sun or shade and most soils. First flowering shoots should be cut down when they wither to stimulate healthy new growth (this surplus material can be used for mulching during dry weather provided the ground is well soaked first). To propagate, cut thick roots into pieces 4in long, place in drill and cover with 3–4in of good soil. In spring young leaves can be confused with those of comfrey *(Symphytum officinalis),* which are edible. Alkanet leaves should not be eaten because they may contain poisonous alkaloids. The surface leaf hairs are softer than those of comfrey, giving a slight shine. Later in the year, comparison of the flowers will avoid any error.

**Uses:** a red dye, extracted from alkanet and its close relative *Anchusa officinalis,* is included in a list of simples used by Hippocrates, the father of medicine, who practised his skills four hundred years before the birth of Christ.

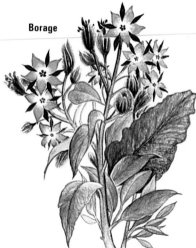
Borage

### BORAGE
(Burrage)
*Borago officinalis*

A hardy annual, sometimes biennial, covered with stiff hairs making it rough to the touch. It has a branching taproot, and the stem grows 20–24in high. The ovate leaves (8 × 4in) are deeply veined, and the vivid blue, starlike flowers have 5 pointed petals, prominent erect black stamens, and a reddish calyx. There is also a white-flowered variety.

**Cultivation:** easily grown where it is required to flower from spring-sown seed, but does not transplant well. Usually produces robust self-sown seedlings in subsequent years.

**Uses:** for those who find cucumber indigestible, borage gives flavour without causing discomfort. If the hairy skin is peeled from young stalks, the succulent inside may be chopped into salads. The flowers are also edible, and are used with the small leaves to give a cool flavour to summer drinks. The beauty of its flowers made borage a popular subject for embroidery, sometimes also showing the bees for whom it is a favourite herb. It can be used as a poultice for external inflammation, and may be beneficial if taken as a tea by those with rheumatic tendencies.

### LUNGWORT
(Soldiers & Sailors, Jerusalem Cowslip)
*Pulmonaria officinalis*

A hardy herb dying down in winter; early in spring dense basal growth shoots from the creeping rootstock. The ovate leaves (6 × 3in) and the stems (to 12in) are hairy and rough to the touch. The foliage shows irregular white blotches and the flower stalks often display blooms of two colours at the same time, deep pink to red and purple or blue. The cowslip-like tubular flowers ($\frac{1}{2}$in) are arranged in short terminal cymes.

**Cultivation:** autumn is the best time to lift and divide roots, thereby avoiding disturbance when the plant is coming into flower in spring. The roots, from which young leaf growth can be seen shooting, should be cut into 3in pieces. Trim off the old leaves and plant in a fairly moist, semi-shady position.

**Uses:** in the 16th century a theory known as the Doctrine of Signatures was expounded by the herbalist and physician , Paracelsus, contending that plants are marked in particular ways in their colour or form to indicate how they are beneficial. The spotted lung-shaped leaves of lungwort pointed to its use for diseases of the lungs and the Latin name *Pulmonaria officinalis* (official herb for pulmonary complaints) established it until recently as a treatment for certain chest ailments. It also served as a pot herb and as a vegetable.

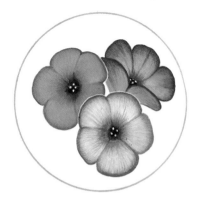

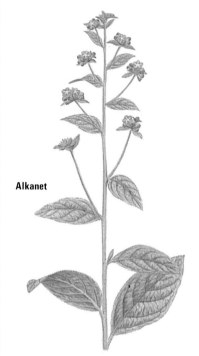
Alkanet

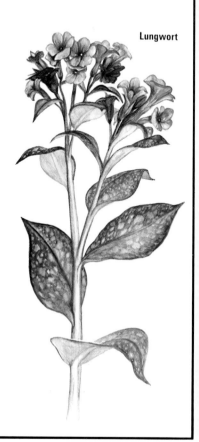
Lungwort

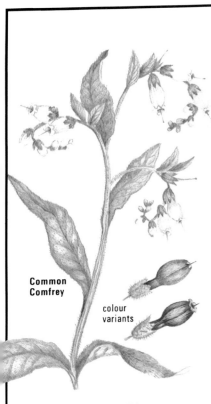

**Common Comfrey**

**colour variants**

## COMMON COMFREY
(Knitbone, Bruisewort)
*Symphytum officinalis*
A strong-growing hardy perennial dying down in winter. The plant (20–40in) develops from the basal leaf growth up squared and flattened hollow stems with pointed ovate deeply-veined leaves decreasing in size from 16 × 6in at ground level to $1\frac{1}{2}$–$2\frac{1}{2}$in under the flower clusters. Leaves are alternate and the bell-shaped tubular flowers, in bloom late spring to autumn, are arranged on one side of the stem. They are usually creamy-white but pink and mauve variants exist.

**Cultivation:** it is so easy to increase comfrey from root cuttings that it is not worth trying to grow it from seed. In spring and autumn roots may be cut into short pieces, laid horizontally in drills and then covered with 2–3in of good soil. Because comfrey produces so much leaf growth it does best in deep moist soil.

**Uses:** Comfrey is a valuable plant which has proved its worth over hundreds of years. Its common names reflect its reputation for helping bones to knit and soothing bruises. The root contains allantoin which encourages healthy cell growth, mucilage which soothes, protein (unusual in plant material) and vitamin B12. The root or leaves, crushed and applied as a poultice, will usually relieve external inflammation and may be taken as a tea to ease internal inflammation. Comfrey ointment applied to burns, sprains and strains, bruises and aching limbs will often give quick relief, but the rough hairy leaves should never be applied directly to the skin because they can act as an irritant. The peeled roots chopped into chunks and the young leaves cooked like spinach make acceptable vegetable dishes.

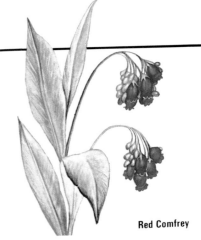

**Red Comfrey**

## RED COMFREY
*Symphytum rubrum*
This crimson-flowered hybrid is not very robust and should be grown in soil containing plenty of humus so that it does not dry out. It needs moisture so a position in semi-shade is best. It seldom grows to more than 12in and comes into flower later than the other comfreys, from July onwards. It is not invasive and will flower on into the autumn attracting attention by the rich colour of its blooms.

**Cultivation:** this less-common and attractive comfrey is propagated, like the others, by root cuttings, but it is worthwhile starting them off in boxes of good compost and taking care to protect the young shoots from slugs. Take the same precautions when the plants are moved to their permanent site.

**Uses:** a good plant to grow near lungwort in semi-shade, providing colour later in the season.

## Family Cannabaceae

### HOP
*Humulus lupulus*
Perennial with stout rootstocks which sends up tender shoots each year. These become tough twining stems (known as bines) which are capable of climbing to a considerable height. Male and female are different plants. The male produces loose panicles of tiny green flowers, while the female flowers are enclosed in round or oval papery yellow-green bracts known as strobiles ($1\frac{3}{4}$in in length). The rough textured leaves are heart-shaped and lobed with toothed edges, the upper leaves are smaller and sometimes without lobes.

**Cultivation:** from seed or suckers taken from strong female plants in spring. To produce good-sized hops the plant requires deeply-dug and well-manured soil. The plants can be trained as decorative climbers in a sunny airy position; the old bines should be cut out after the hops have matured to avoid tangled growth when the new shoots grow from the rootstocks the following spring.

**Uses:** Henry VIII forbade brewers to use the hop in ale, describing it as 'a wicked weed that would spoil the taste of the drink and endanger the people'. At that time it was thought to induce a state of melancholy. Herbs such as alecost, yarrow and wormwood were added to ale for their bitter or aromatic flavours, and the use of hops to give taste and to preserve the beverage was only later acquired from the Dutch and Germans and their name for it 'beer' adopted. A simple home brew can be made by putting 55gr (2oz) hops in 2.25 litres ($\frac{1}{2}$ gallon) boiling water for 15 minutes. Strain, then dissolve 0.45kg (1lb) brown sugar in the liquor. To this add 4.50 litres (1 gallon) of cold water and 2 tablespoonfuls of fresh yeast. Allow to stand for twelve hours and then bottle. Tea made from 2 or 3 hops and a teaspoonful of honey in a cupful of boiling water is a good tonic and sedative. Also hop leaves may be dried, crushed and added, half and half, to Ceylon or Indian teas. In spring tender young shoots, no more than $4\frac{1}{2}$in high, can be picked, tied in bunches and cooked like asparagus. Small muslin bags stuffed with dried hops can be slipped into a pillowcase to help sufferers from insomnia, and in the past the khaki dyes needed for army uniforms were also made from hops.

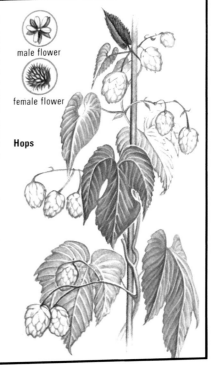

male flower

female flower

**Hops**

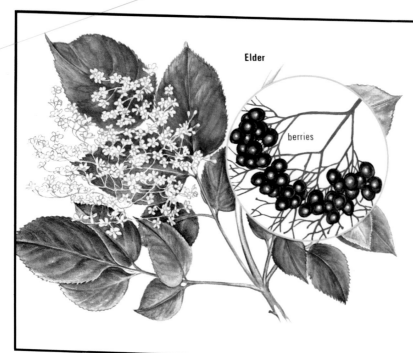

Elder

berries

## Family Caprifoliaceae

### ELDER
(Pipe tree)
*Sambucus nigra*
A large deciduous shrub or small tree (30–40ft) distinguished by its flat heads of creamy flowers in June and purple-black berries in autumn. The dull green leaves, arranged as 5 leaflets with serrated edges, take on a pinkish tinge when the berries ripen.
**Cultivation:** strikes easily from hardwood cuttings pulled off with a heel in spring, cut to 6in and inserted 3in into sandy compost. The tree does well on heavy soil.
**Uses:** few small trees have so much folklore connected with them; Mother Elder was said to protect the garden and its occupants, and in parts of the country people are still reluctant to cut down an elder. Around 400 BC, the elder was included in Hippocrates' list of important plants and it has been in constant use up to modern times for such diverse purposes as children's pea shooters, musical pipes, wines, conserves, cosmetics and cures.

## Family Caryophyllaceae

### CHICKWEED
(Starweed)
*Stellaria media*
A persistent common annual herb with weak sprawling stems which are hairy on one side only. The pale green pointed oval leaves grow in opposite pairs, almost hiding the tiny white flowers ($\frac{1}{4}$in) which have 5 deeply cleft petals and narrow sepals of the same length making a star formation. The fruits are projected on elongated drooping stalks.
**Cultivation:** if allowed to grow on a small damp unwanted piece of ground it will seed freely, propagating itself throughout the year.
**Uses:** it is easy to underestimate a plant most gardeners regard as a troublesome weed, but this herb will provide tasty salad material, even in winter, with a slightly salty, nutty flavour. If it grows in abundance it may be cooked like spinach as a vegetable: wash the leaves and cook in just the water adhering to them, adding a knob of butter and boiling in a covered saucepan over a gentle heat for 5–7 minutes. Before serving, grate a little nutmeg or finely chop some chives over it. Chickweed has a cool soothing effect on the skin and is crushed and applied fresh as a poultice or used in ointments for burns, rashes and to ease the pain of aching joints. It is a favourite food of small birds; because of its ability to propagate itself, the seeds provide valuable winter feed for them.

### SOAPWORT
(Latherwort, Bouncing Bet)
*Saponaria officinalis*
A hairless perennial with spreading rootstock. The stiff, smoothly-ridged stems (20–30in) are pale green, sometimes with a red tinge. The oval pointed leaves (2–3in) with ribbed

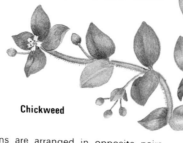

Chickweed

veins are arranged in opposite pairs growing from swollen leaf joints. The pink flowers are either 5-petalled and single or many-petalled and double. Enclosed in a tubular calyx, they grow in terminal clusters in late summer and have the sweet clove scent typical of the pink family.
**Cultivation:** Soapwort does not grow reliably from seed but may be easily propagated in spring from pieces of creeping root showing young leaf buds. Damp friable soil will encourage growth and the name Bouncing Bet reflects the freedom with which the plants grow in a favourable situation.
**Uses:** this plant has served as a natural soap, probably for thousands of years, for cleansing woollens, silks and many beautiful fabrics. In modern times its gentle cleansing action has been successfully used to freshen and restore the colours of old tapestries.

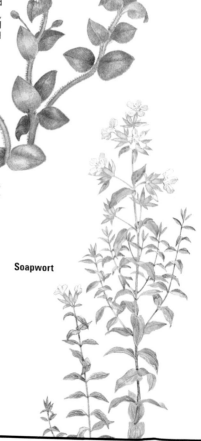

Soapwort

## Family Chenopodiaceae

### GOOD KING HENRY
(Mercury)
*Chenopodium Bonus Henricus*
A hardy perennial herb with taproots and stems (to 20in) bearing dark green, stalked, arrow-shaped leaves, the undersides mealy to the touch. The flowers are dense spikes of tiny green blooms and as the seed ripens the spikes bend into the shape of a crook.

**Cultivation:** by seed sown in spring or late summer or by cutting old roots into pieces retaining a bud or growing point; this can be done in spring or autumn. The established plants will seed freely.

**Uses:** a rather unattractive looking plant but it is rich in iron and is a nutritious cut-and-come-again vegetable. When it is coming through in spring the young growth can be blanched by covering it with a pot or bucket – the tender pink shoots are good in early salads. Later, as the uncovered herb grows, the leaves should be picked frequently, and flower stems should be cut out as they appear, otherwise the leaves become small, coarse and bitter. If seeds are wanted, leave one plant to grow on, flower and ripen seed.

### FAT HEN
(Goosefoot, Lambs Quarters)
*Chenopodium album*
A prolific annual herb (to 30in) found on roadside dumps and field verges. The erect branching stems bear grey-green leaves, oval or arrow-shaped, and mealy on the undersides. The insignificant green flowers grow in short dense spikes from midsummer.

**Cultivation:** by seed; it will grow in poor soil but given better conditions it makes stocky healthy plants.

**Uses:** this plant is rich in iron, calcium, vitamins B1 and C, and has been a valuable source of food since pre-historic times. It is a member of the same family as cultivated spinach, but more nutritious. Like Good King Henry, it should be cut frequently to produce a good growth of leaves. In the past the seed was ground and used as flour, and the plant gets its name of fat hen from being fed to poultry to fatten them. The young stalks are succulent and tender when cooked but they get rather tough when fully grown.

### ORACH
(Arrach, Mountain spinach)
*Atriplex hortensis*
A hardy annual appearing in late spring. The branching stems (28–40in) have stalked, opposite, arrow-shaped leaves with toothed edges, which feel mealy to the touch. The flowers are in red spikes, and the round flat seeds, encased in bracts, are red at first, changing to biscuit-brown when ripe.

**Cultivation:** the plant grows easily from seed but it is best sown in the place it is to grow as it does not transplant well. It will respond to good soil and make much bushier plants than in poor soil.

**Uses:** Orach is notable for the rich beetroot colour of its stems and leaves and it can look very striking grown with grey and soft green foliage plants. The leaves are almost transparent and if it is planted where sunlight can shine through them it adds to its beauty. It may be cooked, like spinach, in very little water; the red colour comes out of the leaves leaving a green vegetable.

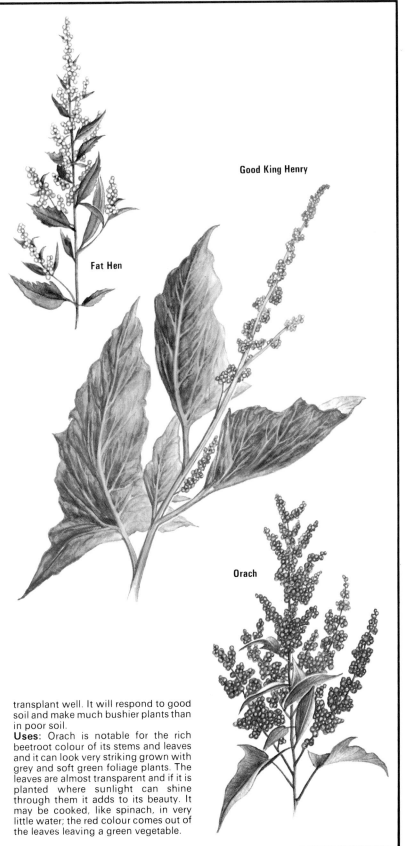

Good King Henry

Fat Hen

Orach

## Family Compositae

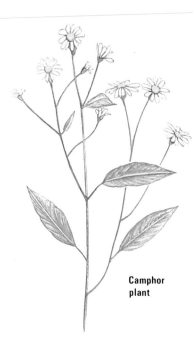

Camphor
plant

common name for burdock, Happy Major, may have originated from the burs being used as buttons to transform, in imagination, a child's plain clothing into a smart-looking uniform.

**Cultivation:** if burdock is introduced into the garden it should be kept apart from any designed herb planting as it seeds freely and will become invasive. If required for edible or medicinal use, it is best planted in a deep, well-drained soil in which it will produce good straight roots.

**Uses:** this plant was included in Hippocrates' list of useful plants. It has been found to contain antibiotic substances which aid resistance to infection and can help to cure skin com-

plaints. A decoction is made from 1-year-old roots which have been washed and scraped. Chop 30gr (1oz) of root and add to 0.85 litre (1½ pints) of cold water which is slowly brought to the boil then allowed to simmer until it reduces to 0.5 litre (1 pint). The mucilage in the root will slightly thicken the decoction which can be drunk and also used to bathe the skin. In spring, country people whose diet had been deficient in vitamins over the winter months used to make a drink made from burdock and dandelion roots which acted as a blood purifier and cleared up skin troubles. The very young stalks may be peeled and chopped into salads and later can be cooked as a vegetable.

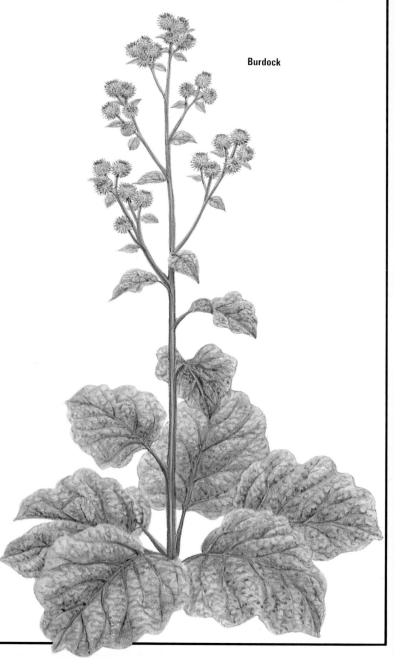

Burdock

## CAMPHOR PLANT
*Balsamita vulgaris*
Camphor is similar to alecost in all its growing habits, but may be distinguished by the colour of its leaves which are a greyer green and its flowers, like small daisies, with white ray florets and yellow disc floret centres.

**Cultivation:** the same as alecost.

**Uses:** the camphor plant smells strongly of camphor oil which comes from the tree *Cinnamonum camphora*. Put among linen, furs and woollens its familiar mothball smell discourages moths. But it can also be dried and mixed with lavender and southernwood, in equal quantities, to make a sweeter-smelling mixture. It is one of the less common herbs.

## BURDOCK, COMMON &
## BURDOCK, GREATER
*Arctium minus & Arctium lappa*
These sturdy biennials share the same characteristics of large downy leaves and round heads of burs. The strong taproots penetrate deeply into the waste ground where the plants are often seen growing wild and the stiff branching stems grow to 28–36in. The coarse textured leaves, sometimes over 12in long at the base of the plant, are arranged alternately and decrease in size up the stem. They are broadly ovate and pointed at the tips, with downy undersides. The leaves of the greater burdock are rounder at the tips and the stalks are furrowed on the upper surface. The egg-shaped buds open to show purple florets, which, together with shorter, sepal-like, hooked bracts, form the burs in late summer. One

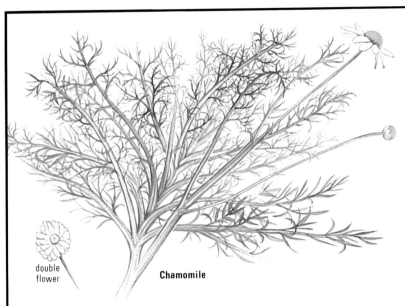

double
flower

**Chamomile**

shape of the leaves, some of which grow 10–12in across, which gives the plant its name. The flowers, like small dandelions (1in), are borne singly on reddish scaly fleshy stems. They appear in spring before the leaves, hence the name Son-before-Father.

**Cultivation:** can be grown from seed gathered from the flower 'clocks' or from pieces of root detached from a plant. Coltsfoot is a vigorous, rampant grower and should be confined to waste patches in the garden.

**Uses:** one of the most valuable herbs for coughs and chest complaints. It is an important ingredient of the herbal tobacco smoked by sufferers from respiratory disorders and can be made into a soothing drink for troublesome coughs.

## CHICORY
(Succory)
*Cichorium intybus*
A perennial with a parsnip-like taproot and a stiff rather hairy stem (20–40in). The leaves first form a rosette at the base of the stem, then diminish in size, deeply cut like dandelions, alternately up the stem. The unstalked flowers are usually in pairs, with ray florets only. They are bright sky-blue in the mornings but fade from midday.

**Cultivation and uses:** easily grown from seed thinly sown out of doors in late spring; the Witloof variety is best for salads. Plant the seedlings 3in apart in a circle and cover them with a large plastic bucket to blanch the leaves. Green unblanched leaves are coarse, woolly and bitter. To force chicory for winter salads, set the plants in rows and earth them up like potatoes in September, ensuring that the ridge is at least 6in over the trimmed crowns of the roots. Magdeburg chicory produces good roots which can be dug, scraped, roasted in shallow trays in the oven and then ground as a coffee substitute. The rather bitter flavour can be neutralized by adding honey.

## CHAMOMILE
(Ground Apple, Roman chamomile)
*Chamaemelum nobile (Anthemis nobilis)*
Chamomile plants can have single, double or no flowers. It is perennial, prostrate or low-growing, with short fibrous spreading roots. The bright green leaves are very finely divided and the plant has a pleasant apple scent, especially when bruised or trodden on. Single flowers have a yellow disc and white ray florets, double flowers are cream-coloured and the yellow disc is not evident.

**Cultivation:** single-flowered chamomile can be grown from seed in spring. Sow the tiny seeds very thinly in boxes or trays and prick out the seedlings when they are big enough to handle. The young plantlets should be set 6in apart in their permanent positions. This is an economical method of raising a quantity of plants, but if they are used for lawn-making quite frequent mowing will be necessary to prevent them becoming straggly. Double flowered chamomile should be propagated by pulling off young rooted plantlets from the parent at the end of May or in September. Non-flowering chamomile, now known as 'Treneague', is the best one to make into fragrant paths, small lawns or a mossy looking 'mat' in front of a garden seat or around a sundial, bird-bath or other garden ornament. The young plantlets should be set out on clean ground 6in apart in staggered rows and made very firm. They will spread out, filling in the spaces between them. Rolling helps to establish the new roots and all weeds should be removed by hand as soon as they appear; selective weed-killers will destroy the chamomile. When the lawn is established it will need mowing a couple of times during the summer to keep it compact and stimulate new growth.

**Uses:** one of the most beneficial of

herb teas, chamomile was recommended for headaches, chills, fevers, digestive trouble, as a fomentation for swellings, for nervous conditions and as a tonic to brighten fair hair. For a pint of chamomile tea allow 6 flowers, infuse for 5–10 minutes and, if liked, add a small teaspoonful of honey to each cup.

**Coltsfoot**

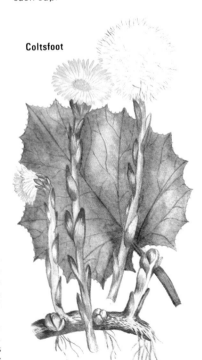

## COLTSFOOT
(Son-before-Father)
*Tussilago farfara*
Herb with creeping rootstock and net-veined, broadly heart-shaped leaves with edges toothed and undersides covered with cottony down. It is the

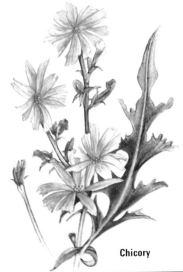

**Chicory**

## DANDELION
(Lion's tooth, Priest's crown)
*Taraxacum officinale*
A common, widely distributed perennial herb with a strong taproot. The irregularly jagged toothed leaves in the basal rosette vary in shape and are lanceolate with a grooved central vein which directs rain to the root through the centre of the rosette. The flowers, borne singly on hollow stems, are

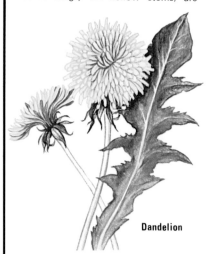

**Dandelion**

composed only of ray florets maturing to the familiar dandelion 'clock', whose windborne seeds, each with its own parachute, ensure continuity.
**Cultivation:** by seed sown in spring. If bigger, less toothed leaves are wanted, it is possible to obtain seed of a cultivated variety of dandelion. All dandelion leaves are slightly bitter, the young ones less so, but much of the bitterness can be removed by blanching. This is done by covering the plants to exclude the light with large flat stones, strong lightproof boxes, flower pots, plastic buckets or sheets of black or blue polythene. Precautions should be taken to prevent slugs eating the succulent blanched growth.
**Uses:** the dandelion is one of the most valuable of all known herbs, having more uses and medicinal properties than many cultivated vegetables. Dandelion coffee made from roots washed, scraped, roasted and ground, is the best substitute for true coffee. The white latex juice from the roots and stems was used in the treatment of warts and moles. The leaves contain vitamins A, B and C. Not only are they good in salads but help to stimulate the appetite, act as a mild laxative, are an effective diuretic, and provide relief from dyspepsia, liver disorders and some rheumatic conditions. The herb is safe to take in any quantity. Dandelion wine is one of the best-known country wines.

## FEVERFEW
(Featherfew)
*Chrysanthemum parthenium*
Hardy short-lived perennial with many branching stems coming from the fibrous root and forming a compact bushy plant (18in high and about the same across). The lime green leaves (2–3in), composed of pinnate leaflets ($\frac{1}{2}$in), have serrated edges. The single flowers, which have a yellow disc and white ray florets, $\frac{1}{2}$–$\frac{3}{4}$in across, bloom from summer to autumn. Cultivated feverfew, or bachelors' buttons, has creamy-white double flowers with ray florets ($\frac{1}{2}$–1in).
**Cultivation:** feverfew grows freely from seed and will flourish in sun or shade on shallow well-drained soil; the seed can be sown in spring or early autumn. Plants grown from seed of the double variety may revert to single flowers. At most times of the year, when the weather is suitable, cuttings can be pulled off with a 'heel' from the base of the plant and set in sandy compost.
**Uses:** the names feverfew and featherfew may be corruptions of 'febrifuge', a term used to describe a herb employed to treat chills and fevers. When feverfew is found wild it is often near old cottages or in farmyards as it was thought that it could purify the atmosphere and help to ward off infection. An infusion of the leaves or flowers was taken to cure nervous headaches, to improve digestion and as a general tonic. Modern research has established the value of feverfew in the treatment of migraine. It is recommended that three leaves should be taken daily in a sandwich or chopped and added to food. It may also be of benefit in the treatment of some arthritic conditions.

## GOLDEN ROD
*Solidago virgaurea*
An erect perennial with a dense growth of smooth or slightly hairy stems coming from rhizomes. Varies in size from 2in on rocky or cliffside areas to 36–40in on hedgebanks or dry open woodland. The lanceolate finely-toothed leaves are arranged alternately up the stems. On the upper part of the stem, branching flower stalks spring from the axils of the leaves and form a terminal panicle of small golden yellow flowers (4in across) with a few disc and ray florets. The lower part of the flower is encased in green sepal-like bracts.
**Cultivation:** from pieces of rhizome pulled off at soil level in spring and set in good compost. Golden rod is particularly responsive to the quality of the soil in which it is grown and has a pleasant fragrance when it blooms from midsummer into autumn; it is a vigorous grower and should not be allowed to spread too far.
**Uses:** as its generic name which comes from *solidare* (to consolidate or make whole) indicates, golden rod has a reputation for healing wounds when applied as a poultice or used as an infusion to bathe the wound.

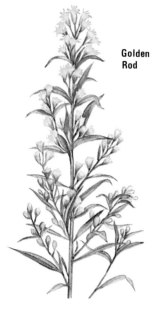

**Golden Rod**

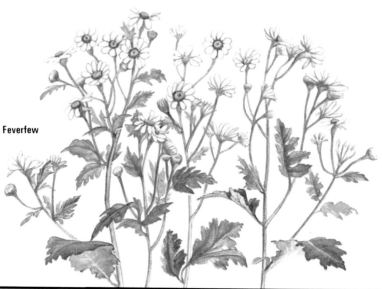

**Feverfew**

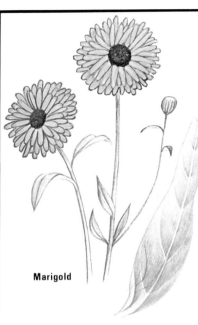

**Marigold**

# MARIGOLD
(Pot Marigold)
*Calendula officinalis*
A hardy annual (up to 20in) familiar in many gardens because it seeds freely year after year. It has a fleshy white taproot and juicy stems branching at angles, with stalkless, lanceolate, slightly hairy leaves (up to 6in) which are sticky to the touch. The single orange flowers have disc and ray florets up to 4in across. In bloom for much of the year, its Latin name *calendula* testifies to its presence 'throughout the months'.
**Cultivation:** marigolds germinate quickly from spring sown seed. Seed sown in autumn will survive in poor conditions, but spring sowing makes healthier plants on good soil. Allow at least 12in between each seedling so that the plants have room to develop if a good crop of leaves and flowers is to be harvested for drying. The hard curved seeds, sometimes $\frac{1}{2}$in long, look curiously like petrified grubs. The flowers will come into bloom in quick succession and need picking every day or so. The outer ray 'petals' (florets) are stripped off the disc, spread thinly on sieves and placed in a warm place in the dark (see page 4), the petals should be lightly tossed with the fingers every day to ensure even drying, and then stored in air-tight containers out of the light. In this way, they will keep their bright orange colour.
**Uses:** Calendula has an ancient history and has proved of considerable importance in the treatment of many skin complaints because of its antiseptic and anti-inflammatory properties. Both leaves and flowers are used and affected parts are bathed with an infusion or dressed with an ointment or lotion made from the plant. The juice can be expressed from the leaves and applied directly to the skin. It is used for ulcers and other inflamed areas and can be taken internally as a tea. The flowers yield a good orange dye which one of the old herbalists suggests was once used to colour the hair of those 'not content with the colour God had given them'. The name pot marigold has nothing to do with the plant being grown in a pot but is a corruption of the word 'pottage', indicating its use in soups and stews. It makes a wholesome colouring agent for cheese, and the young leaves and flowers are used in salads and are a good substitute for saffron in rice for buns and cakes.

# SOUTHERNWOOD
(Old Man, Lads Love)
*Artemisia abrotanum*
A woody perennial losing its leaves in winter. It forms a shrubby bush (to 40in) which from spring through to late autumn is densely covered with fine thread-like leaves. The flowers are sometimes absent or so inconspicuous as to be hardly noticed but the aromatic smell from the foliage has made this herb a long time favourite cottage garden plant.
**Cultivation:** like many of the artemisias, southernwood does not grow well from seed in Britain but cuttings strike easily if taken in spring or late summer. It should be trimmed into shape each autumn to prevent the bushes getting straggly and ungainly.
**Uses:** this was one of the strewing herbs of olden days. When walked on, its wholesome scent helped to make unhygienic conditions more supportable. It was also given to children to expel worms, and put among clothes to discourage moths (which is the reason for its French name of garderobe). An infusion rubbed into the scalp was thought to stimulate the growth of hair. Rubbing any infusion on a hairless head will not make hair grow, but the massaging of the scalp with some herb infusions will have a healthy effect on existing hair. Dried southernwood can be added to pot pourri mixtures to give a lemony scent. Mixed with lavender or any of the fragrant mints and oatmeal, and made up in small muslin or cotton bags, it can be hung under the hot water tap to give fragrance to a bath and help to soften hard water.

# WORMWOOD
(Old Woman)
*Artemisia absinthium*
A woody perennial (to 36in). The basal leaves are lobed and deeply divided; the stem leaves are linear. All are covered with close silky hairs on their upper and lower surfaces, which gives the plant a silvered look. The flowers develop on the terminal and lateral stems as panicles of small yellow rayless blooms which look rather like mimosa.
**Cultivation:** from seed or cuttings in spring or late summer. The seed is minute and should be mixed with fine sand and the whole scattered thinly on top of the soil and not covered. There is a cultivar, Lambrook Silver, which makes more compact and dense silvery growth than the type and is the better one to grow in a herb bed. It should be propagated by cuttings or root division.
**Uses:** in the past, wormwood was administered to get rid of intestinal worms. An infusion made from it is drunk to settle a disturbed stomach, but the flavour is so intensely bitter – it is one of the bitterest herbs known – that it is not found acceptable by most people.

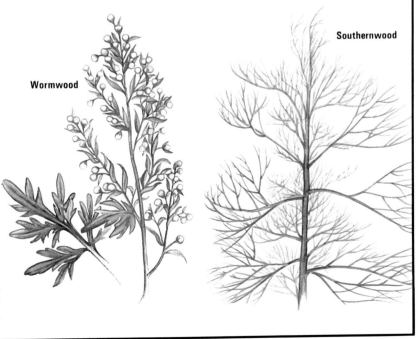

**Wormwood**

**Southernwood**

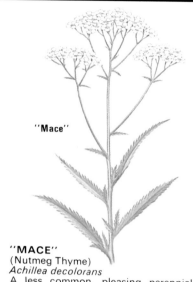

"Mace"

## "MACE"
(Nutmeg Thyme)
*Achillea decolorans*
A less common, pleasing perennial herb (to 14in) which dies down in winter. Fibrous roots form a clump from which grow stems bearing alternate linear fine-toothed leaves (2in). The flowers are in terminal clusters with creamy-white ray and short disc florets ($\frac{1}{2}$in across).

**Cultivation:** from division of root in spring when small pieces may be easily separated from the parent plant. It likes a well-drained sunny position and the clumps should be split and replanted every 3–4 years.

**Uses:** the true mace is the webby aril around the nutmeg which is marketed as blade or ground mace. This herb gets its names of 'mace' and 'nutmeg thyme' because its smell is so similar to the true spice and it can be used instead of nutmeg or mace in cooking.

## SNEEZEWORT
*Achillea ptarmica*
A bushy erect perennial (to 24in) dying back in winter with dense stem growth and dark green, lanceolate, serrated leaves (3in). It has clusters of true white double daisy-type flowers with ray florets and an insignificant central disc. Flowers from midsummer, opening a succession of flower clusters until autumn – a good foil for other colours.

**Cultivation:** by division of root in spring or autumn. Likes a rather moist position and will spread steadily. The root becomes densely entangled so it is wise to divide the clumps and replant every 3–4 years.

**Uses:** the name sneezewort indicates its use, when dried and powdered, as a snuff taken to clear the nasal passages.

## SUNFLOWER
*Helianthus annuus*
A well-known annual producing plants from 20in to 16ft high. The round, rough erect stems carry ovate leaves (2–12in) with toothed edges, and the solitary flowerheads, with golden ray and brown disc florets, can be anything from 3 to 12in across.

**Cultivation:** from seed sown in pots or boxes indoors in April. The young plants must be put out when all danger of frost is past, or sown out of doors in May where they are to grow. The flowerhead is top heavy so support will be needed and a sheltered site is advised. Thought to be a native of Mexico this plant has been grown in many parts of the world as a valuable domestic and commercial commodity, the seed providing food for humans and animals, the leaves used for cattle food, the stem fibre employed in paper-making. Sunflower margarine is among the best of those high in poly-unsaturates and sunflower oil is an excellent substitute for olive oil in salads and cooking or herb oils for skin treatment.

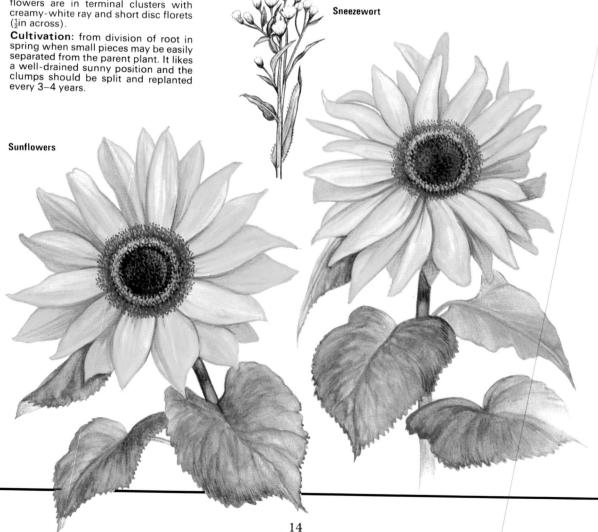

Sneezewort

Sunflowers

## TANSY
(Buttons)
*Tanacetum vulgare*
An erect hardy perennial (to 48in) on stiff stems with dark green, feathery, pinnate, irregularly toothed leaves, which are strongly aromatic. The flowers are corymbs of gold 'buttons', all disc florets, from midsummer.

**Cultivation:** by root division or pieces of rhizome pulled off in spring or autumn. Tansy, a vigorous herb to the point of becoming invasive, is best in an informal setting.

**Uses:** tansy cakes and tansy puddings were eaten during Lent and the herb is thought to have been one of the bitter herbs of the Passover. Bitter it certainly is and should be used with discretion in cooking. It excels at discouraging flies, and as it is often found by riversides can help fishermen to keep flies away from themselves and their catch. A few fresh leaves rubbed between the hands to bruise them and then tucked into clothing gives protection from flies when working or sitting in the garden. Bunches cut freshly each day, bruised and laid across open windows, help to keep flies away from the house, but the herb is only effective while fresh and aromatic. For a spray against aphids, boil 220gr ($\frac{1}{2}$lb) tansy shoots in 1 litre of water for 10 minutes. Cool, thoroughly strain, add a couple of drops of washing up liquid and use within a day or so. Do not store.

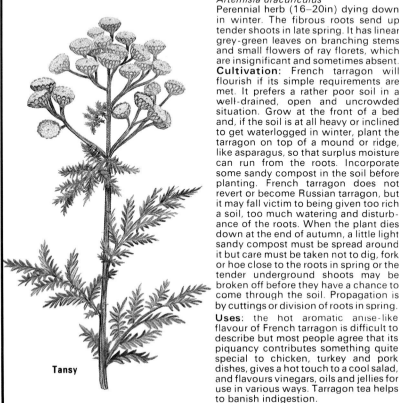

Tansy

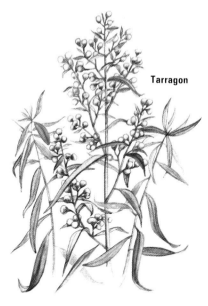

Tarragon

## TARRAGON, FRENCH
(Little Dragon)
*Artemisia dracunculus*
Perennial herb (16–20in) dying down in winter. The fibrous roots send up tender shoots in late spring. It has linear grey-green leaves on branching stems and small flowers of ray florets, which are insignificant and sometimes absent.

**Cultivation:** French tarragon will flourish if its simple requirements are met. It prefers a rather poor soil in a well-drained, open and uncrowded situation. Grow at the front of a bed and, if the soil is at all heavy or inclined to get waterlogged in winter, plant the tarragon on top of a mound or ridge, like asparagus, so that surplus moisture can run from the roots. Incorporate some sandy compost in the soil before planting. French tarragon does not revert or become Russian tarragon, but it may fall victim to being given too rich a soil, too much watering and disturbance of the roots. When the plant dies down at the end of autumn, a little light sandy compost must be spread around it but care must be taken not to dig, fork or hoe close to the roots in spring or the tender underground shoots may be broken off before they have a chance to come through the soil. Propagation is by cuttings or division of roots in spring.

**Uses:** the hot aromatic anise-like flavour of French tarragon is difficult to describe but most people agree that its piquancy contributes something quite special to chicken, turkey and pork dishes, gives a hot touch to a cool salad, and flavours vinegars, oils and jellies for use in various ways. Tarragon tea helps to banish indigestion.

## YARROW
(Staunchweed, Soldiers Woundwort)
*Achillea millefolium*
A hardy perennial found growing wild on roadside verges, with creeping rootstock and finely cut leaves (2–4in), each segment deeply indented giving a feathery effect. Basal leaves are stalked, those on the stems stalkless and shorter. Stems grow to 20–24in and bear corymbs of dull white, pinkish and sometimes deep pink disc and ray florets, the flat heads 2$\frac{1}{2}$–3in across, which flower throughout the summer.

**Cultivation:** pieces pulled off at soil level, usually already rooted, will 'take' with no difficulty and spread rapidly.

**Uses:** the common names of this herb show that it was used as a styptic, a plant to stop bleeding. The generic name *Achillea* came from the legend that Achilles staunched the bleeding wounds of his soldiers with yarrow; the specific name *millefolium* describes the finely cut 'thousand leaves' of its growth. In less hygienic days than these a cobweb was placed over a wound to arrest the blood flow and help it to coagulate; the fine network of yarrow leaves might well achieve the same result. Taken in combination with elderflower and peppermint, fresh or dried, it is a favourite herbal infusion to be drunk at the first signs of a cold. A cool infusion of leaves used as a cosmetic wash is good for greasy skins, while the young basal leaves may be chopped into salads. Used as an activator, yarrow will help to break down garden rubbish for compost.

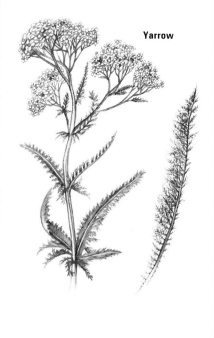

Yarrow

## Family Cruciferae

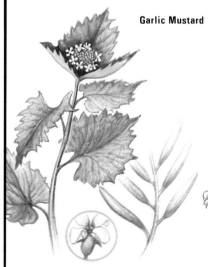

**Garlic Mustard**

### GARLIC MUSTARD
(Jack-by-the-hedge)
*Alliaria petiolata*
A biennial with an erect stem (12–36in). The fresh green, stalked, heart-shaped leaves have toothed edges, and release a strong garlic smell when bruised. The small white flowers, which appear in spring, have 4 petals in cross formation and are arranged in a corymb. Garlic mustard can be found growing wild under hedgerows and in waste places.
**Cultivation:** by seed in late spring. The plant will self-sow when the seeds ripen late in the following spring or early summer and then die.
**Uses:** the young leaves used sparingly will give a garlic flavour to salads and other dishes and may be chopped into sauces (as the common name 'Sauce-alone' suggests). The plant has anti-septic properties and the juice is used to cleanse ulcers and skin eruptions. The leaves crushed until moist may be rubbed on to aching limbs to promote a feeling of warmth.

### HORSERADISH
*Armoracia rusticana*
A hardy perennial herb cultivated by the ancient Egyptians and probably for centuries before their civilization. From the long tapering taproot (20–24in) basal leaves grow to 20in. Lanceolate with indented edges, and with a prominent midrib on the underside, the coarse leaves are often mistaken for docks. The flowering stems, bearing small leaves, terminate in small clusters of tiny 4-petalled white flowers.
**Cultivation:** pieces of root with a bud attached should be cut off in spring and planted in good deep soil. Horseradish spreads rapidly and must be kept to a part of the garden where it cannot become a nuisance. Every few years it is wise to dig up the old bed and replant.
**Uses:** best known as a sauce served with roast beef, but it is also good with fish. Home-made horseradish sauce is much hotter than that commercially produced. An infusion of a little scraped horseradish root with honey added may help to soothe a persistent cough; and a gentle massage with the cut root will help to warm stiff or aching joints.

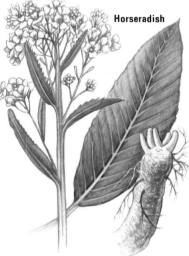

**Horseradish**

### LADY'S SMOCK
(Cuckoo flower)
*Cardamine pratensis*
This is one of the prettiest of spring wild flowers and welcome as a garden plant. Its name, cuckoo flower, associates it with the time the cuckoo returns to Britain, but the plant is widely distributed in northern Europe. It is a slender erect perennial (8–16in) first showing a rosette of pinnate leaves with rounded leaflets. The stem leaflets which then appear are narrower; and the flowers, arranged in a raceme ($\frac{1}{2}$–$\frac{3}{4}$in), are 4-petalled and mauve-pink with darker mauve veining in the petals (occasionally double flowers occur).
**Cultivation:** from seed sown in spring. The plant does best in damp places and will grow in semi-shade.
**Uses:** like many so-called 'weeds' this plant has many virtues. It is rich in vitamin C and was a welcome blood-purifying herb in the spring when scurvy was an annual problem after winter months of food lacking necessary vitamins. Of the same family as watercress it makes a good substitute for it, as well as for mustard and cress. Good in salads and soups.

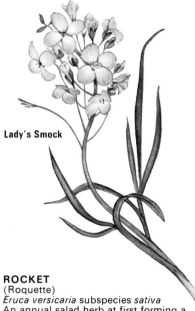

**Lady's Smock**

**Rocket**

### ROCKET
(Roquette)
*Eruca versicaria* subspecies *sativa*
An annual salad herb at first forming a rosette of dark green deeply-lobed leaves from which the purplish flower stem rises 8–20in with narrower leaves and reddish flower buds opening to show 4 narrow petals with purple-brown veins (1in).
**Cultivation:** it likes a moisture retaining soil in an open sunny position. Seed should be sown in succession from late spring to enable one to take tender young leaves from the quickly growing plants – the older leaves soon get coarse.
**Uses:** a salad herb with a cress flavour.

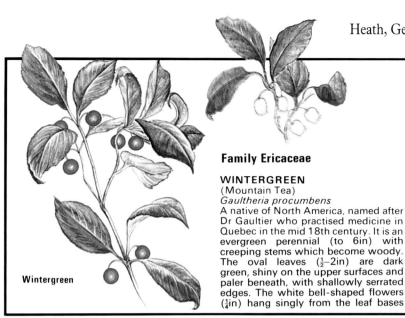

Wintergreen

## Family Ericaceae

### WINTERGREEN
(Mountain Tea)
*Gaultheria procumbens*
A native of North America, named after Dr Gaultier who practised medicine in Quebec in the mid 18th century. It is an evergreen perennial (to 6in) with creeping stems which become woody. The oval leaves ($\frac{1}{2}$–2in) are dark green, shiny on the upper surfaces and paler beneath, with shallowly serrated edges. The white bell-shaped flowers ($\frac{1}{4}$in) hang singly from the leaf bases and bloom from midsummer, maturing to red berries in autumn.
**Cultivation:** by cuttings or division of root in spring or seed (berries) in autumn. It is a member of the heather family and likes a lime-free peaty soil.
**Uses:** the leaves when bruised or broken off give off a warm aromatic smell familiar to those who remember having their chest rubbed for coughs and colds. The oil is employed in a 'rub' used externally for rheumatic and muscular pains and to flavour dental preparations. A few leaves may be infused to make an aromatic tea. Wintergreen is a good ground cover plant for semi-shady areas or to grow between shrubs like rhododendrons or azaleas which need a lime-free soil. The genus includes many small, low-growing, spreading shrubs which may be cultivated for the interest of their foliage, flowers and berry fruits.

## Family Gentianaceae

### CENTAURY
(Centre of the Sun)
*Erythraea centaurium*
An annual with yellowish fibrous roots and erect square stems (to 12in). It has light green, oblong basal leaves and opposite, stalkless stem leaves which become narrower as they reach the terminal branching clusters of bright pink tubular flowers, coming into bloom at midsummer. The name centaury is thought to have come from the Centaur Chiron, famed in Greek mythology for his skill in the use of medicinal plants; attention was first drawn to the herb because of his claim that it had cured him of a wound from a poisoned arrow.
**Cultivation:** from seed sown in spring on the surface of the soil in a sunny well-drained position. The plants will self-sow but do not like being transplanted.
**Uses:** the herb is bitter to taste but it is a good simple tonic, will stimulate a reluctant appetite and helps the digestion. This is a delightful small herb which can be grown in a rockery or trough garden and will naturalize between paving or gravel.

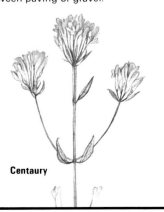

Centaury

## Family Guttiferae

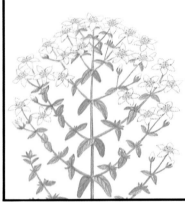

### ST JOHN'S WORT
*Hypericum perforatum*
A stiff-stemmed perennial (20–24in) with dense creeping rootstock. The light green leaves are oblong, linear and opposite, and there are terminal cymes of golden-yellow flowers which have 5 petals and many stamens. The leaves and petals are dotted with oil glands. In bloom towards the end of June for St John's Day, the plant was dedicated to the saint, but it was being used medicinally long before his time.
**Cultivation and uses:** may be grown from seed in spring or division of root in spring or autumn; it likes an open position and light soil. It yields a red oil used externally to treat aching joints, wounds and burns, which is thought to be antibiotic and antiviral.

## Family Iridaceae

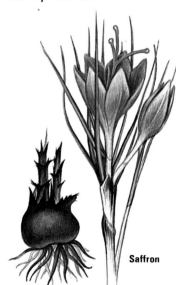

Saffron

### SAFFRON
(Saffron Crocus)
*Crocus sativus*
A perennial similar in appearance to the spring-flowering crocus. The corm produces narrow grass-like leaves in late summer followed by purple flowers with prominent branching styles.
**Cultivation:** a good rich soil is required for the corm to produce flowers, and plants should be at least 4in apart. The styles bearing the stigmas are the parts of the flower collected for drying and well over 4000 are needed to yield an ounce.
**Uses:** this scarce, highly-valued herb was greatly esteemed for its colour and perfume by the poets of ancient times. At one time it was grown commercially in England and the town of Saffron Walden testifies to the area having been well suited to its cultivation. Nowadays true saffron is used for colouring and flavouring rice, buns and cakes or can be taken as a tea for digestive troubles or as a light sedative. Care must be taken not to confuse saffron with the poisonous *Colchicum autumnale*.

## Family Labiateae

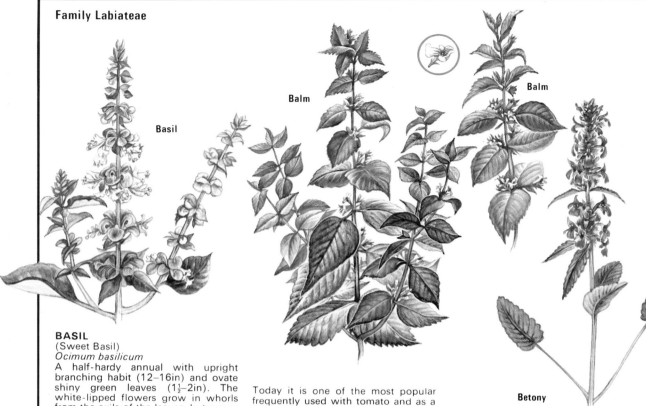

Basil

Basil

Balm

Balm

Betony

### BASIL
(Sweet Basil)
*Ocimum basilicum*

A half-hardy annual with upright branching habit (12–16in) and ovate shiny green leaves (1½–2in). The white-lipped flowers grow in whorls from the axils of the leaves, but are an insignificant part of the plant. When any part is bruised, the characteristic clove-like scent is evident. Bush basil *(Ocimum minimum)* grows as a smaller compact bush with leaves only ½–¾in. Opal basil *(O. basilicum purpurascens)* has the habit of sweet basil, with beautiful purple leaves and a pink flower.

**Cultivation:** all the basils are half-hardy in this country and the seed should not be sown out of doors before June. It can be sown indoors from late April but the young plants must not be planted out until mid-June, or when all danger of frosts and cold nights is over. In a good summer it will do well in a warm, well-drained, sheltered border, but it may be wise to keep some plants indoors if the weather is uncertain.

**Uses:** basil is a herb of contradictions – its flavour is much sought after by many, but others find it quite unacceptable. In the past many legends have grown up around it. The Greeks thought it signified hatred and poverty and that it grew best when the seed was sown accompanied by curses and abuses, but in Italy it was given as a love token. In the past, some people believed that no foods could be eaten from a plate under which a sprig of basil had been placed, while others claimed that it 'procured a cheerful and merry heart'. Keats wrote a long poem about Isabella who buried her lover's head in a pot of basil; in Egypt women scattered basil on the graves of their loved ones.

Today it is one of the most popular frequently used with tomato and as a herb to flavour oils and vinegars.

### BALM
(Lemon Balm, Bee Balm)
*Melissa officinalis*

A hardy perennial growing into dense clumps (to 36in). The square stems bear ovate leaves with crenate edges (2–3in) growing in opposite pairs. The insignificant flowers, primrose-yellow in bud, open to white from midsummer.

**Cultivation:** by seed sown in spring or division of root in spring or autumn. Established plants self-sow freely, and the progress of balm through the garden will have to be controlled as young plants appear in unexpected places.

**Uses:** the refreshing lemon scent of this plant, although not evident before the leaves are bruised, makes it one of the favourite herbs to grow today, as it has been for thousands of years. Its name *Melissa* is derived from the Greek word for bee leaf; beekeepers used to grow the herb for the nectar it yields and rub it on their hives to attract swarms. The name 'balm' suggests its use as a mild sedative. An infusion made from the fresh leaves is a delicious summer drink, taken either hot or iced, which will act as a digestive after a meal. The fresh young leaves add a delicate lemon flavour to any dish and are good in salads, with fish, in banana sandwiches, and with other fruit. The leaves rolled into a ball to release the oil may be used to soothe stings and midge bites. The herb needs careful drying to preserve its scent and flavour and should be removed from its drying place as soon as it is crisp and then stored in an airtight container.

### BETONY
(Wood Betony)
*Stachys officinalis (Betonica offic.)*

Perennial herb with some basal growth persisting through the winter. It has fibrous roots and the stems grow from a rosette of stalked leaves (to 12–20in). The stem leaves, slightly hairy, are oval with crenate edges. The rosy-purple flowers appear first in whorls coming from the axils of the leaves and then as a dense terminal spike.

**Cultivation:** can be grown from seed sown in spring or late summer, or from rooted plantlets eased out of the parent plant in spring. It prefers a semi-shady position and is a pleasing-looking herb with its rosette of shapely leaves in spring and spikes of flowers in summer.

**Uses:** quite extravagant claims have been made in the past for the medicinal and magical powers of betony. An infusion made from the herb will in fact act as a mild sedative to quieten anxiety or soothe headaches, and it is also useful as a good bitter tonic drink and, externally, for cleansing and helping to heal wounds. The dried leaves can be included in herbal smoking mixtures and are an ingredient of some snuffs.

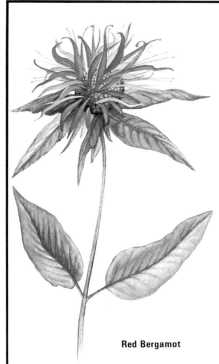

**Red Bergamot**

# BERGAMOT
(Oswego Tea)
*Monarda didyma* and cvs
Herbaceous perennials dying down in winter and spreading out from the parent plants by rhizomes. The stems are square, erect (14–40in) with slightly serrated ovate-lanceolate leaves in opposite pairs arranged alternately up the stem. The decorative whorled flowerheads show a random display of narrow, tubular florets with deeply cleft lips and visibly protruding stamens. There are crimson, scarlet, purple, lavender, pink and white bergamots but the most fragrant is *M. didyma*.
**Cultivation:** from seed sown in late spring or, to ensure true progeny from the parent plant, from rhizomes pulled from the outside of the plant in spring or early autumn. Bergamot is closely allied to the mints and likes the same conditions: a moist humus-rich soil with some shade during the hottest part of the day. After about three years the plants should be lifted, the original heart of the plant discarded and the healthy outside growth split into new clumps and replanted; if this is not done the plant loses its vigour and is inclined to die out. Young growth should be protected from slugs.
**Uses:** *M. didyma* has a delicious scent similar to the bergamot orange *(Citrus bergamia)* from which it gets its name and which yields the bergamot oil used in commerce. The lavender-coloured *M. fistulosum*, abundantly wild in North America where it is a native, is the Oswego Tea commonly drunk by the American Indians which became

famous when it was adopted as a beverage by many Americans after the Boston tea party to demonstrate their protest against the tax imposed on imported tea. The white-flowered bergamot 'Snow Maiden' is not as common or robust as the other cultivars but its purity of colour and refreshing lemon scent are worth seeking. The early-flowering 'Croftway Pink' is thyme scented. Young bergamot leaves may be used in salads and fresh or dried for tisanes. It is interesting to note the subtle changes of flavour that are evolved by blending the leaves with 'ordinary' tea. Bergamot holds its scent well when carefully dried and is a valuable ingredient for pot pourri.

# BUGLE
(Sicklewort, Carpenter's Herb)
*Ajuga reptans*
A perennial herb with spreading stolons sending up erect stems (4–6in). It has opposite pairs of leaves which are oblong and stalked at ground level, and oval and stalkless on the stems, which terminate in a spike formed by several whorls of flowers. These are blue-lipped with purple-blue bracts between the whorls, giving the whole a densely packed appearance.
**Cultivation:** the stolons root freely and it is possible to detach pieces with plantlets already formed at the nodes. Each plantlet will throw out rooting stems, so this herb makes an excellent ground cover plant where speed of growth is welcome.
**Uses:** the herb is bitter and astringent and for many centuries has had a reputation as a styptic and wound herb; its common names of sicklewort and carpenter's herb indicate its use in stopping the bleeding of cuts caused by accidents with tools.

# CATMINT
*Nepeta faassenii (Nepeta mussini)*
A hardy perennial dying down in the winter. In spring it sends up softly hairy grey-green serrated leaves (1in) which form clumps of dense bushy growth 10–12in tall and 20–24in across. The flowers grow on long arching spikes and are a soft misty lavender blue.
**Cultivation:** catmint can be grown from seed sown in spring or division of root clumps in spring or autumn. It likes a well-drained soil and sunny position, and will come into flower in late spring. When the flower stalks have died off they should be removed, and the bush trimmed into a neat shape so that the foliage will give pleasure until it sends up a second crop of flowering stems. In late autumn about half the length of flowering stalks should be cut back, leaving some to give protection during the winter to the rootstock which is susceptible to damage from hard frosts and cold east winds. This protection will be increased if the plants are surrounded with a dressing of compost, leaf mould or peat. In spring, when the young shoots can be seen to be growing, the rest of the old growth should be removed. Your cat, or indeed any others in the neighbourhood, will find it a most desirable place in which to curl up on sunny days, to the detriment of the shape of the bushes:
**Uses:** this is a favourite border plant because it makes a good low hedge and gives much the same misty blue effect as lavender. It has a strange scent, which is difficult to describe and not to everyone's taste, but as a decorative herb it has much to commend it.

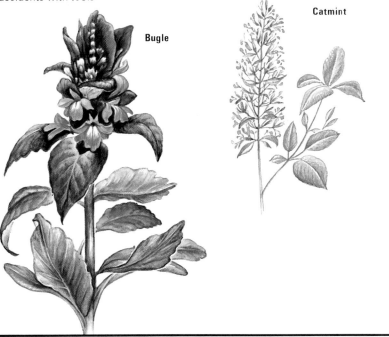

**Bugle**

**Catmint**

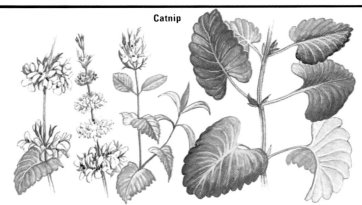

Catnip

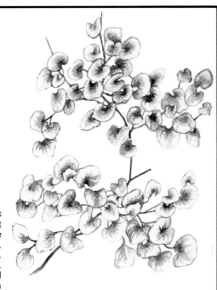

Curled Golden Marjoram

## CATNIP
(Catnep)
*Nepeta cataria*
This plant is best treated as a biennial as it has a habit of dying during the winter after flowering, particularly on heavier soils. It has not the attractive appearance of catmit, looking more like nettle or balm and growing upright (to 36–40in). The ovate leaves have crenate edges and are in opposite pairs and in their axils whorls of small white-lipped flowers with purple dots appear.
**Cultivation:** on a light soil catnip grows easily from seed sown in spring or will self-sow from ripe seed in late summer. It is irresistibly attractive to cats and will need to be protected from them. There is an old saying:

'If you set it the cats will eat it,
'If you sow it the cat's won't know
  it.'

– in other words the sowing of seeds gives no smell of the herb but if it is handled for planting and the leaves or stems are bruised and release the smell, cats seem to come from miles around and will roll on it, eat it and in the end destroy it. If one is fond of cats this is definitely their herb and the dried leaves can be stuffed into pseudo 'mice' as playthings for them.
**Uses:** this is the medicinal catnip and the fresh or dried herb is used as an infusion for many minor complaints such as headaches, indigestion, colds, colic and diarrhoea. It may have a useful function in the garden as a spray against plant pests, using at least 55gr (2oz) fresh herb to 0.55 litre (1 pint) of water. Legend has it that chewing the root of catnip makes timid people brave and there is an account of a reluctant hangman who used to eat it to help him carry out his gruesome task.

## HYSSOP
*Hyssopus officinalis*
A woody perennial herb making a bush 24in tall and 20in across when in flower. The stems are branched and the linear, entire leaves ($\frac{3}{4}$–$1\frac{1}{2}$in) are stalkless. The bright gentian-blue lipped flowers grow in whorls from one side of the stem forming a spike.
**Cultivation:** hyssop can be grown from seed sown in spring or early autumn. Pink hyssop *(H. officinalis*

*rosea)* and white hyssop *(H. officinalis alba)* may also be grown from seed but their progeny may revert back to the blue type. To ensure that the pink, white or blue colours are reproduced, propagation should be from cuttings, best taken in spring. Hyssop does well in most soils but likes a sunny position and after flowering it should be cut back to a good shape. It responds well to this trimming which prevents it becoming too woody and tending to break away from the centre of the bush. The blue, pink or white hyssops make good low hedges and if kept regularly trimmed will last for many years; they become a mass of flower spikes giving a wonderful show of colour, rather like large heathers.
**Uses:** there have been differences of opinion as to whether the hyssop mentioned in the Bible was *Hyssopus officinalis* or one of the marjorams or the caper plant. Hyssop has a clean, wholesome smell reminiscent of cough medicines and a tea made from it can be soothing for a troublesome cough. The oil from the flowers and leaves has antiseptic properties and may help to soothe bruises and aching joints. It has also been used in perfumery and liqueurs. Hyssop helps to stimulate the appetite and tender young leaves can be added to salads or soups.

## CURLED GOLDEN MARJORAM
*Origanum aureum crispum*
A neatly-growing small herb with fibrous roots. The stems are erect (to 10in) with kidney-shaped crinkle-edged leaves that are bright gold during the summer. As the strength of the sun decreases, the leaves tend to become less golden and in the winter they are green. The small clusters of flowers may be pink or white.
**Cultivation:** this marjoram responds to a sunny position, as do other members of the family, but as it is less robust than other perennial relatives it should be given light soil, or heavy soil made light for its benefit. It is a charming little plant and one of the smaller herbs suitable for a trough garden.
**Uses:** it can be eaten or used for a tea but its interesting crinkly golden foliage is so attractive it is a pity to cut it off.

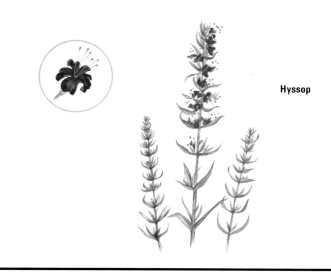

Hyssop

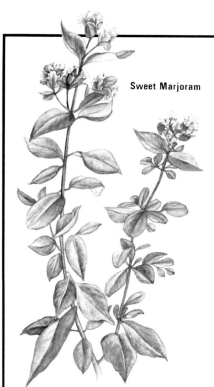

Sweet Marjoram

## SWEET MARJORAM
(Knotted Marjoram)
*Origanum marjorana*
In warm climates this herb can be classed as a perennial but in Britain it is best treated as a half-hardy annual as it does not survive cold conditions out of doors. Growing on fibrous roots it forms an erect branching plant (8–12in), with elliptical grey green opposite leaves (to 1in) and spherical flower buds looking like tight knots, from which it gets its name 'knotted marjoram'. The insignificant small white flowers arranged in a corymb are in little clusters. The noteworthy feature of this marjoram is its delicious warm aromatic fragrance which prompted one of the herbalists of old to say that it 'should be given to those suffering from overmuch sighing'. Its scent is so good it *must* have a cheering effect!

**Cultivation:** from seed sown indoors in late April or May, or outside in June when all danger of frost is past. It needs a well-drained light soil and a sunny sheltered position with no over-crowding.

**Uses:** this lovely little herb can be made into a refreshing fragrant tea which is also good as an aid to digestion or as a mild expectorant for coughs. It is good with salads, tomato or egg dishes, in pizzas and freshly chopped as a garnish for cream soups, courgettes and avocado dishes. Like many herbs it is best added to cooked dishes just before serving as overcooking spoils its flavour. The dried herb is an excellent ingredient for pot pourri or to hang in muslin bags under the hot water tap of the bath. When travelling in hot weather take a few sprigs for its refreshing scent.

## OREGANO
(Wild Marjoram, Origano)
*Origanum vulgare*
A compact low growing perennial with fibrous roots. The densely growing erect stems, sometimes reddish, make a bushy plant (to 18in) and, like the pointed ovate dark green leaves (1in), are hairy. The small pinkish-purple flowers are arranged in corymbs and bloom from midsummer to autumn. Wild marjoram is found on warm sunny banks, cliff-tops and rocky areas limestone districts.

**Cultivation:** it can be grown from seed but as the marjorams are apt to hybridize it is wise to start with plants of the true *Origanum vulgare*. At certain times of the year the different marjorams can look much alike but they each have characteristic scents and if one can get to know these, identification is made easier. The aroma of oregano is sweet, round and warm. Established plants can be split into small clumps in spring and replanted in quite poor soil; the less lush the plant grows the more intense is the flavour.

**Uses:** a pleasant tea is made from oregano which will settle a disturbed stomach or help to ease a headache. The herb is used in many meat dishes, with pizzas, pastas, salads and soups, and associates well with mushrooms.

## LAVENDERS
One of the best known and loved of all the herbs, grown in many gardens where no special thought has been given to herbs as such. *Lavandula vera* ('true'), *L. spica* ('spike') and *L. officinalis* ('the official one') have evolved as two main types – *L. angustifolia* (narrow-leaved) and *L. latifolia* (broad-leaved) – but there are many hybrids and cultivars. Popular lavenders include Old English (*L. angustifolia*), Dutch or Grey Hedge (*L. latifolia*) and Munstead (*L. angustifolia*).

**Cultivation:** all lavenders are bushy perennials and most are hardy. Originally from warm Mediterranean countries, they like as sunny a position as possible and if the garden is exposed to east wind they will appreciate some shelter. The soil should be well drained and compost or manure dug in at planting, and then as a mulch in autumn, to encourage good growth and flower production. If the soil is deficient in lime, a dressing should be given in spring.

**Uses:** lavender for drying should be cut when about half the blooms on the spike are expanded otherwise some may discolour or drop before all are in bloom. It is easier to rub the dried blooms off the stalks if all the flower-heads are kept facing one way. A small posy of lavender spikes pressed now and then to release the oil is an effective insect repellent. The florets can be used in salads and tisane made from lavender, fresh or dried, is a pleasant mild sedative. Lavender oil has many commercial uses in perfumery.

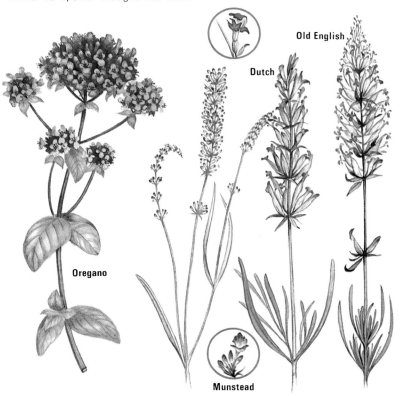

Oregano

Old English

Dutch

Munstead

## MINTS

The genus Mentha is one of the most interesting groups of herbs, differing in size, habit, marking, colour and smell to such an extent that it may be difficult to believe that they all belong to the same family. Indeed it has been said that the mints pose more problems of identification and classification than any other genus of comparable size. Anyone who has grown mint over a number of years may have noticed that plants which could once be turned into a delicious mint sauce somehow lose their flavour, become rank and may no longer look exactly the same as when first planted. A mint bed grows vigorously at first and then has a tendency to become an overgrown tangle of roots all competing for nourishment. It is a greedy plant and to do well needs a rich moisture-retaining soil. Because it grows so fast when first planted, taking advantage of all available nourishment in the soil, do not feed it if you want to restrict its growth and stop it spreading. It may be put in a bottomless bucket or have tiles sunk around it to restrain it, but it will still escape or, if it exhausts the soil and becomes too dry, it will start to deteriorate. The plant grows and spreads by rhizomes, shallowly rooting stems which probe out in all directions for food. If it is to be kept growing healthily in one place, all the old growth should be dug and discarded at least every three years, and the ground replanted with strong young rhizomes taken from the outside of the parent plants. Dig some good compost into the soil at the same time. If the variegated-leaved cultivars are grown for their colour effect in herb beds, one has to be ruthless in carrying out the same procedure, otherwise the rhizomes will creep through the bed, coming up in the middle of other subjects and defeating the object of the original planting scheme. Most of the mints have evolved from the native cornmint

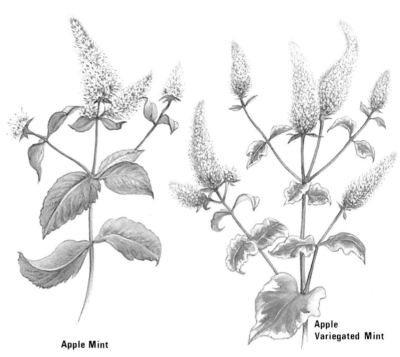

**Apple Mint**

**Apple Variegated Mint**

(*M. arvensis*), water mint (*M. aquatica*), apple mint (*M. suaveolens*) and the naturalized spearmint (*M. spicata*). From these parents have come innumerable hybrids and back to them many mints to some degree revert.

**Cultivation:** all mints are perennials. It is difficult to ensure that those grown from seed will come true and to be certain of this they should be propagated by division of rhizomes in spring and autumn, planting into a good moisture-retaining soil. If any sign of deterioration or reversion is detected the roots should be dug up and burnt.

### APPLE VARIEGATED MINT
*M. suaveolens variegata*

Growing to 24in it has prettily marked leaves with white edges or white blotches on the outsides of the leaves. Sometimes entirely white shoots appear. It is a decorative plant for the garden and as a pot plant drapes well over the edges of the pot. The scent is good and it can be used for cooking, mint tea or dried for sweet bags or pot pourri. Always propagate from runners which are producing well-marked foliage.

### APPLE MINT and BOWLES MINT
*Mentha suaveolens* and *M. suaveolens rotundifolia* var. *Bowles*

These are two very similar species and are sometimes confused as the Bowles mint is often listed as 'Apple' mint. Their erect stems (to 36in) have hairy, grey-green leaves which are both opposite and alternate. The flowers are in dense whorls forming a rather blunt spike. The leaves of Bowles mint are round, to 3in long and 1½in broad. Both these mints have a good flavour with a fresh apple undertone. Bowles mint is very hardy, sometimes surviving a mild winter without dying back, and is more rust resistant than other mints. For sauce, mint jelly or tea either of these mints are excellent and one should not be discouraged from using them because of the hairy appearance of the leaves. The flavour of all mints gets stronger and sometimes rank in a dry season, when the plant is in flower. If it is cut back tender new growth will soon appear.

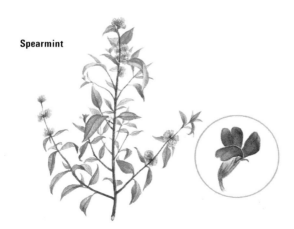

**Spearmint**

## PINEAPPLE MINT
*M. citrata cv.*

A handsome mint growing with a rather spreading habit and much-branched stems (30–50cm). The striking yellow and green striped leaves are ovate and shiny, with a fragrance which, if not exactly like pineapple, is certainly fruity. The rhizomes branch freely and are noticeably whiter than some of the other mints. If it is ruthlessly kept within bounds this is a colourful mint, particularly in spring before the plant develops flowering shoots with their short round heads. It can be employed as a ground cover plant where its spreading habit is welcome. After flowering, towards the end of summer, if it looks a bit tatty, cut off the ragged growth and it will grow again, looking attractive until it dies down for the winter.

variegated apple mint. When crushed the leaves have a gingery smell and this becomes a pleasant fragrance when the herb is dried for adding to pot pourri. Ginger mint is also used as a herb tea.

## PEPPERMINT
(Black Peppermint)
*M. x piperita*

One of the most important commercial herbs, yielding peppermint oil for flavouring and medicinal purposes. The plant grows to 24in with erect, reddish stems and bronze-red pointed, shiny leaves ($1\frac{1}{2}$–3in) with serrated edges. Flowers in leaf axils and short tapering spikes. There is no mistaking this mint as true peppermint has a strong smell familiar to everyone. Peppermint tea may be taken for digestive complaints, colds (especially when combined with

yarrow and elderflower), hot as a warming beverage, or iced as a clean tasting, refreshing summer drink. If peppermint leaves are crushed and frequently smelled, the 'fumes' from them can help to clear blocked nasal passages. To make delicious after-dinner mints, carefully select some good peppermint leaves, wash and gently dab dry, then brush with lightly beaten white of egg and dust on both sides with icing sugar. Lay the leaves on a cake rack and place in a cool oven to dry and become crisp. Store, when cool, between sheets of greaseproof paper in an airtight container. Pineapple mint leaves, borage, violet and primrose flowers, and red rose petals can quickly be preserved this way. Some peppermint leaves kept in a screw-topped jar of sugar will, like vanilla pods, impart their flavour to the sugar which can then be used in confectionery or baking. White peppermint has green, slightly hairy leaves with coarser serration, but there is little difference in the smell and both are cultivated for the production of oil.

## CORSICAN MINT
(Spanish Mint)
*M. requienii*

A prostrate mint forming a close mat with a mass of dull green heart-shaped leaves (to $\frac{1}{4}$in) and tiny purple flowers, each smaller than a pinhead. The whole plant has a pepperminty smell. On light soils it makes a good carpeting plant in semi-shady areas and on a heavier soil seems to do well in shade or full sun and survives most winters. After severe winters when it seems to have succumbed, it will re-emerge in spring, obviously from self-sown seed. Small clumps will soon spread and can be lifted with soil attached, split and replanted in May or September. It can be walked on with no ill effect and grown between paving, in gravel, rockeries or sink gardens. The tiny flowers, some of the smallest known, give a purple flush to the foliage when in bloom. Though a native of Corsica, *M. requienii* has become naturalized in the United Kingdom and in Ireland.

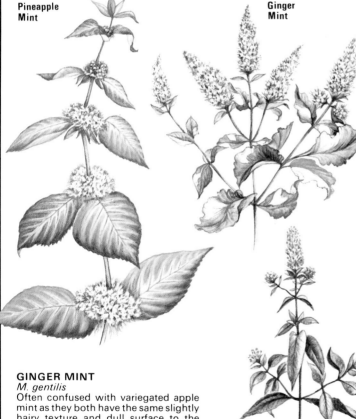

Pineapple Mint

Ginger Mint

## GINGER MINT
*M. gentilis*

Often confused with variegated apple mint as they both have the same slightly hairy texture and dull surface to the leaves. Whereas variegated apple mint has distinctive white edging to the leaves, ginger mint, although variable in its marking (sometimes having wholly green leaves, sometimes ones with random cream blotches) has an interesting, clearly defined half-and-half colouring displayed on some leaves, one side of the central vein being green and the other side cream. The cream and green marking becomes more evident as the plant matures. The terminal leaf buds are also a creamy colour, rather than the white of

Peppermint

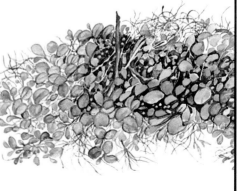

Corsican Mint

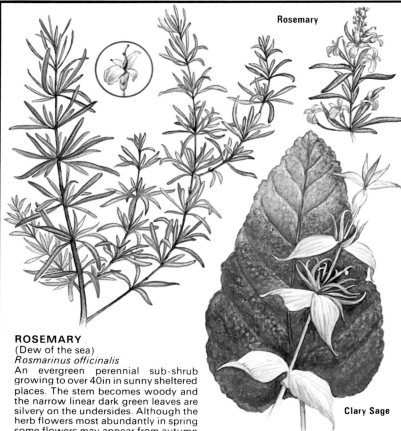

Rosemary

Clary Sage

### ROSEMARY
(Dew of the sea)
*Rosmarinus officinalis*
An evergreen perennial sub-shrub growing to over 40in in sunny sheltered places. The stem becomes woody and the narrow linear dark green leaves are silvery on the undersides. Although the herb flowers most abundantly in spring some flowers may appear from autumn through a mild winter if the shrub is sheltered against a warm wall. The foliage and misty-blue lipped flowers have a strong balsam-like smell which has made rosemary one of the most favoured herbs over many centuries.

**Cultivation:** rosemary may be grown from seed but the resultant plants may not have the same robustness in surviving winter conditions as plants grown from cuttings taken from healthy stock plants. The bulk of rosemary seed is imported from warmer climates where the herb grows abundantly and the progeny may not have the stamina to flourish in colder conditions. However, if this is appreciated and the young plants are protected from frost pockets and east winds they may well acclimatize and become hardier. Rosemary must have a well-drained soil, which is possible even on clay if sand is added, remembering that the plant's natural habitat is in sandy seaside areas.

**Uses:** rosemary oil and waters have been used extensively in cosmetic and medicinal preparations for thousands of years. It has digestive, tonic and antiseptic properties and has been used as a gargle and taken as a tea for nausea, headaches and as a sedative. Externally the oil is used as an embrocation by sufferers from aching joints and neuralgia. Rosemary is also an excellent tonic for the hair. A handful of stems should be put in a jug and boiling water

poured over them. The jug is covered and left to cool and the strained liquid massaged into the scalp and used as a final rinse after washing the hair. As rosemary is evergreen it is usually possible to pick it fresh from the bush, even in winter, so drying is unnecessary. It can be rubbed into and cooked with lamb, pork, chicken and fish. Some sprigs kept in a jar of sugar will impart its flavour for use in apple pies, cakes and biscuits. In winter mulled cider with rosemary and cloves makes a heart-warming beverage for those coming in from the cold. An orange with short tips of rosemary pushed into the skin (a fine skewer will make the holes) and tied with ribbon makes an aromatic pomander-like 'visiting gift'.

### SAGE
*Salvia officinalis*
A familiar perennial herb in most gardens, growing as a bush (to 36in across) with woody rootstocks and much-branched stems bearing oblong grey-green entire leaves with wrinkled surfaces.

**Cultivation:** there are two types of common sage, narrow-leaved and broad-leaved. Narrow-leaved sage is grown from seed and has more pointed, rather greyer leaves than the broad-leaved type which does not produce viable seed and must be propagated

vegetatively. The flowering narrow-leaved sage is decorative, with spikes of purple flowers. Broad-leaved sage produces good crops of leaf for drying; its less intense flavour is preferred for culinary purposes in many cases.

**Uses:** the name salvia, coming from the Latin for 'to save', indicates the virtues attributed to this herb of restoring health and saving from sickness. It was extolled in a proverb: 'He that would live for aye must eat sage in May'. In addition to its culinary use in stuffings, sauces and salads, it can be taken as a wholesome tea throughout the year.

### CLARY SAGE
(Clear Eye)
*Salvia sclarea*
Botanically this handsome plant is a biennial, but if the flower stalks are removed in autumn it will sometimes persist for 3 or 4 years. In the first year it forms a rosette of broad cordate leaves, and in the second year the flowering stems grow to 40–60in, the leaves becoming smaller towards the top. The branching flower spikes are drooping in bud and become erect as the flowers open. The small-lipped flowers, pink-white or purple-white, are insignificant compared with the large pink bracts which give the plant its striking effect.

**Cultivation:** by seed sown in spring or autumn. This plant looks best against a dark background.

**Uses:** clary sage oil is used as a fixative for perfumes. Its common name 'clear eye' may come from the word clary, or more likely from its use to remove obstructions from the eyes. The mucilage from the soaked seeds helps to do this, and to soothe the inflamed eyes. The young leaves dipped in batter were cooked as fritters.

Sage

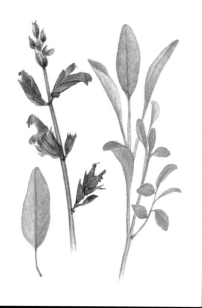

## WINTER SAVORY
(Bean herb)
*Satureja montana*

A small, hardy, evergreen, bushy herb of compact habit (to 12in). The branching stems bear opposite pairs of linear, dark green leaves ($\frac{1}{2}-\frac{3}{4}$in) and from midsummer small white or pale mauve flowers.

**Cultivation:** from seed, cuttings, layering or division. Mountainous regions are savory's natural habitat, so a well-drained poorish soil will suit it and in such a position it will persist for many years if trimmed back into shape after flowering and given a compost mulch in autumn. It should be given plenty of space, not overcrowded by other plants.

**Uses:** as a savoury herb in soups, casseroles and in salads. Blended with a little grated horseradish, it goes well with fish, particularly trout. As we put sprigs of mint with peas, in Europe savory is added when cooking beans for, as its alternative name indicates, it complements all types of beans. This perennial savory is an excellent alternative to the annual summer savory.

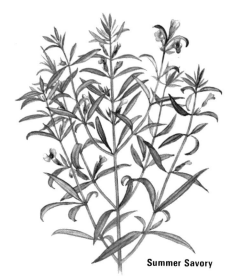

Summer Savory

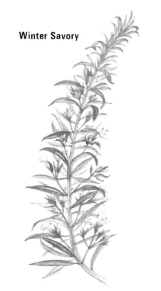

Winter Savory

## SUMMER SAVORY
*Satureja hortensis*

An annual herb with erect, soft, sparsely branching stems (12in) and long internodes. The leaves ($\frac{1}{2}-\frac{3}{4}$in) are light green and there are pale pink flowers in the axils of the leaves.

**Cultivation:** from seed sown indoors in April or outside in May. The plant will not survive frost in spring or autumn. It is one of the annual herbs which respond to being potted and brought indoors in early autumn to keep growth going. If winter savory is being grown from seed it is a good idea to sow summer savory also, so that the annual herb can be used while the perennial plants are getting established. Although the alliterative summer savory is usually the one mentioned in recipes it seems to have little to commend it compared with the perennial winter savory.

**Uses:** the same as for winter savory. Savory vinegar made with wine vinegar is good served with fish or used in salad dressings. It provides a good digestive tea and helps to soothe the irritation from insect bites.

## THYME
(Common Thyme)
*Thymus vulgaris*

A small bushy perennial (to 12in) with much-branched stems becoming woody. There are two types, one with lanceolate grey-green leaves, the other with ovate green leaves (2–3in). In late spring the bushes are covered with masses of flower spikes bearing whorls of purple florets.

**Cultivation:** by seed which usually produces the grey-green narrow-leaved type or by cuttings, layering and division of root from bushes showing the broader green leaves. Thyme needs a well-drained soil and open position

and should be sheared of the dead flowering growth if it has not been cut for culinary or medicinal use. The herb may be cut for drying in May before the flowers open and again in autumn, after which compost should be spread around the plants.

**Uses:** a well-known herb for flavouring stuffings, sausages, soups and salads. It has valuable antiseptic properties as a medicinal herb. An infusion should be drunk for colds, coughs, throat infections and used to bathe skin eruptions.

## SILVER THYME
*Thymus vulgaris* 'Silver Posy

A small bush thyme with attractive silver-edged leaves, the undersides of which are tinged with pink. It grows like common thyme and has the same scent. It should be grown in full sun and trimmed into shape after flowering to prevent the growth becoming straggly. Mulch with compost in the autumn.

## SILVER THYME
*T. citriodorus* 'Silver Queen'

A cultivar with lemon-scented foliage but too prone to revert to its green-leaved parent, lemon thyme. Growing on very poor soil may delay this reversion, but if constant silver foliage is required it is better to grow the reliable 'Silver Posy' which seldom reverts.

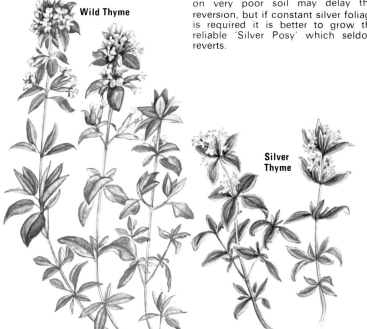

Wild Thyme

Silver Thyme

## Family Lauraceae

### BAY
(Sweet Bay, Noble laurel)
*Laurus nobilis*
A shrub or small tree with dull green or dark red woody stems. The shiny dark green alternate leaves are ovate or broad lanceolate with wavy edges (to 5½in). The plant flowers irregularly with small clusters of unisexual yellowish blossoms appearing in the axils of the leaves in early summer.
**Cultivation:** bay can be grown from seed but it is a long process. It is best grown from cuttings, taken in late summer and potted up in a sharp sand or gritty compost and overwintered in a cold greenhouse (in frost free areas the pots may be sunk into soil under a west wall). Low-growing stems may be layered and pegged down from the parent bush. Young bay trees should be given protection from east winds and in areas where severe winters are expected it is best to grow small trees in tubs or large pots so that they can be brought under cover for winter. With established trees severe weather may damage the top growth but the tree will usually shoot again from the base.
**Uses:** bay trees are used as ornamental feature plants either as natural bushes or trained into various shapes. The aroma of a crushed bay leaf is very pleasant and is used in cooking with fish, lamb, marinades and soups, for bouquet garni and milk puddings. Bay leaves do not retain good colour after drying and if possible fresh leaves should always be used. The noble laurel was a symbol of achievement in ancient times and branches of bay were woven into crowns for victors at the games and to celebrate great artistic successes (hence the term 'poet laureate'). It was thought to have protective and antiseptic virtues and the bruised leaves were smelled or the branches burned where there was infection. Care must be taken not to confuse the leaves of *L. nobilis* with those of the Cherry laurel *(Prunus laurocerasus)* with leaves serrated at the edges, and Mountain laurel *(Kalmia latifolia)* with flowers that look as if they might have been made of piped fondant icing. Both of these plants can be poisonous.

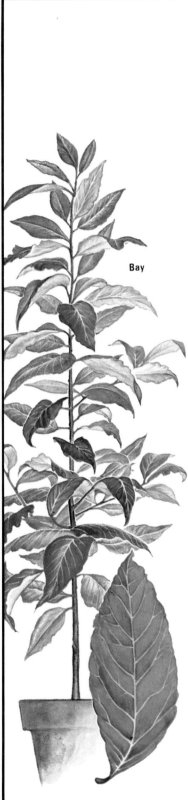

Bay

## Family Linaceae

### LINSEED FLAX
*Linum usitatissimum*
This annual grows on slender stems to about 48in with blue-green, lanceolate, alternative, stalkless, leaves (1–2in). The obovate, 5-petalled flowers are sky-blue and grow in loose terminal corymbs.
**Cultivation:** by seed sown in late spring on good well-drained soil. Flax is best sown where it is to flower as it does not transplant well.
**Uses:** this delicate-looking plant has been an invaluable element in the economy of many civilizations since at least 5000 BC. Cloth spun from flax has been found in ancient tombs. It was used for clothing and hangings in houses and temples; for sails and the thread for fishnets; for ropes and bow strings; and, knotted with tow, stuffed into the cracks of boats. To make cloth, the flax was soaked, dried in the sun, tried into bundles, and then, as a medieval account has it, 'knockyd, beten, rodded and gnodded, ribbed and heklyd and at last sponne'. Equally important is its yield of oil. Commercial crops of linseed have been grown in many parts of the world for use in paints, varnish and putty, as a fattening food for cattle and in veterinary medicine. Externally it may be used as a poultice for boils, inflammation and wounds. There is an annual red-flowered flax *(L. rubrum)* which has rich crimson flowers and blooms over a long period. Sow seed in late spring.

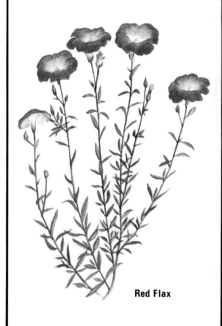

**Red Flax**

## Family Liliaceae

### CHIVES
*Allium schoenoprasum*
An easily-grown perennial herb with fibrous roots and grass-like tubular tapering leaves (6–10in). The leafless flower stems terminate in bunched heads of thrift-like purple florets.
**Cultivation:** from seed sown in spring or autumn or by dividing the clumps into 6–10 bulbs for replanting. It will grow well in most soils and although the plants die down in late autumn they usually reappear with the first mild weather of February. When the seeds are black and ripe in late summer they may be shaken out of the flowerheads and sown in shallow drills. In late autumn pull up some fine soil either side to protect them for the winter.
**Uses:** the tender green leaves of chives give a mild onion flavour. They can be chopped into almost any kind of salad, or used with egg, cheese, fish and vegetable dishes to flavour or garnish.

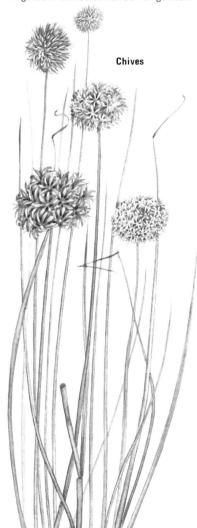

**Chives**

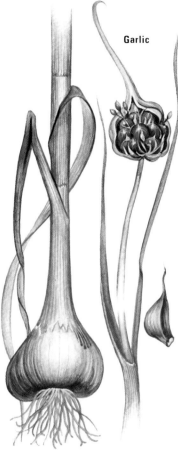

**Garlic**

The newly opened flowerheads are also edible. They may be split into individual florets and added to salads, savoury rice or soups just before serving. Giant chives grows about twice as big as the common chives and the bulbs can be pulled like spring onions. Chives leaves do not keep their flavour and colour as well as other herbs when dried but they freeze well.

### GARLIC
*Allium sativum*
A perennial compound bulb, although usually grown as an annual like onions and shallots. The bulb is made up of many bulblets known as 'cloves' held together within a paper sheath. The leaves are flat and linear, tapering to about 12in. The flower stalk in late summer has a terminal head of white florets and tiny bulbils.
**Cultivation:** cloves separated from the parent bulb should be planted about 4in apart in good, well-drained soil in a sunny position. On light soils planting should be done in autumn, on heavy soils in early spring as soon as the soil can be worked. The bulbs will be ready for harvesting in early autumn.
**Uses:** for thousands of years, the valuable antiseptic properties of garlic have protected people from a number of unpleasant infections. It destroys certain harmful bacteria and is beneficial in combating coughs, colds, bronchial conditions and skin complaints. A cut clove of garlic is an effective first aid remedy pressed on to cuts and scratches. It was an important ingredient of a recipe known as 'the vinegar of the four thieves' which gave immunity to a band of infamous rascals who, at a time of plague in Marseilles, robbed the dead and dying of their valuables. In cooking, garlic enhances many dishes and loses its strong smell. If it gives offence when eaten raw, parsley, mint, sweet cicely or peppermint will help to freshen the breath. It is rich in vitamins and undoubtedly a health-promoting herb.

### TREE ONION
(Egyptian onion)
*Allium cepa* var. *proliferum*
Alliums are rich in the variety they offer and tree onion may be considered an exhibitionist in the group. At the top of sturdy hollow stems (to 20in) heads of small onions develop, usually 4–6 in number. Sometimes another slender stem grows through them, again surmounted with tiny onions. If the first tier is thinned to 4 and secondary growth discouraged, the onions can be used for soups or when only small quantities are needed in cooking. As the plant ripens the stems turn straw-coloured and bend over, setting the young onions at soil level to restart the cycle of growth. These young onions, put several in a pot on a kitchen window sill, will sprout freely and provide winter onion green over a long period. They are more successful than chives, which if treated in this way tend to get thin and wispy.

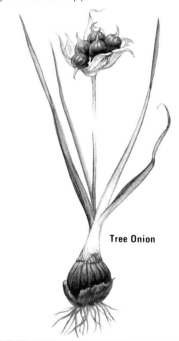

**Tree Onion**

## Family Malvaceae

### COMMON MALLOW
*Malva sylvestris*

A rather straggling perennial herb, either prostrate and spreading or erect and bushy, according to habitat. The basal leaves are palmate and crinkly, sometimes spotted at base, and becoming more deeply lobed on the stems. The flowers have 5 notched petals, rosy-pink with purple stripes, twisted in bud stage and in a hairy calyx. The seeds, or nutlets, are arranged in a flat circular disc. Aptly named 'cheeses' by country children, they are edible and have a pleasant hazelnut flavour.

**Cultivation:** this plant grows readily from seed or by pieces of the rootstock pulled off at the base of the plant and replanted. In the wild it is a low-growing plant found on roadsides and dry banks, but cultivated plants will reach 32–36in in height, making a handsome, bushy plant massed with flowers over a long period.

**Uses:** all mallows have emollient properties and are useful to draw and soothe boils, inflamed areas or un-healthy sores. The tender young stalks can be cut into pea-sized pieces and cooked as a vegetable in spring with mint, chives, savory, lovage or some other flavouring herb as they are rather bland on their own.

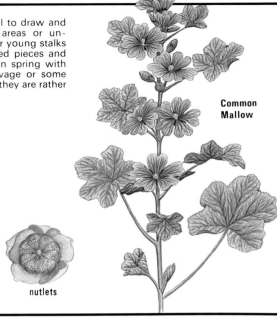

**Common Mallow**

**nutlets**

## Family Onagraceae

### EVENING PRIMROSE
*Oenothera biennis*

An edible biennial which in the first year forms a rosette of elliptic, slightly-toothed leaves and a stumpy taproot. In the second year this sends up a flowering stem (32–40in) which branches and shows reddish colour on the stem and midribs of the lanceolate leaves. Racemes of flowers come from the axils of the leaves. The flower bud is encased in a hairy red calyx which splits to reveal the broad yellow petals, delicately scented in the evenings.

**Cultivation:** from seed sown in spring or autumn. It will grow in quite poor conditions and most soils; and self-sows freely.

**Uses:** the first year leaves can be used in salads while tender and the roots grated and eaten raw or cooked as vegetables. By the time the plant comes into flower the roots are coarse and stringy. Evening primrose is an American native plant and has naturalized in Britain since introduction in the 17th century, and may be found growing wild on roadsides and in seaside areas. From a medicinal point of view it may excite more interest than it has done in the light of modern research into its constituents and their potential for preventing heart ailments.

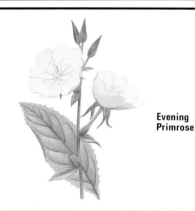

**Evening Primrose**

## Family Polygonaceae

### SORREL
(Sour sauce)
*Rumex acetosa*

A hardy perennial herb with taproot and reddish stems (32–40in) terminating in whorled spikes of tiny red-green flowers, ripening to rich brown seeds.

**Cultivation:** seeds of the broadleaved cultivated sorrel germinate quickly sown out of doors in late spring and plants should not be allowed to flower if maximum leaf is required. It will grow well in most soils and conditions. This broad-leaved type is sometimes called French sorrel, but so also, confusingly, is the small Buckler's sorrel *(Rumex scutatus)* with broad reniform, lobed leaves, which grows only to about 20in. Wild sorrel *(R. acetosella)* is found in open meadows and grassland and recognized by its deeply cut spear-shaped leaves. All sorrels have the sharp apple flavour which is refreshingly thirst-quenching when chewed on a hot summer day and delicious added to salads or used as a sauce, as an alternative to apple sauce, with pork, duck or goose. The sharp flavour is due to the oxalic acids the plants contain and too much should not be eaten by anyone with a tendency to gout or rheumatic complaints. To make sorrel sauce, take a couple of handfuls of leaves, wash and finely chop them, then gently simmer them in the water still adhering to them. To $\frac{1}{4}$ pint (150ml) of the juice that forms add $\frac{3}{4}$ pint (450ml) of stock and a couple of sprigs of chopped sweet cicely. Blend a dessertspoonful of flour with enough cold milk to make it creamy and add this to the herbs and stock, with a knob of butter and a scrape of nutmeg. Bring gently to the boil and stir for 2 or 3 minutes then remove from the heat and if possible put through a blender or liquidiser.

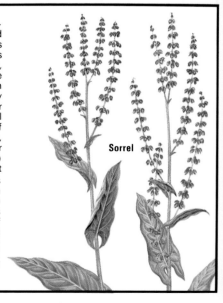

**Sorrel**

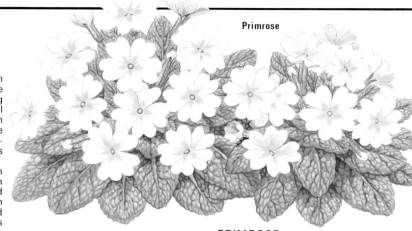

**Primrose**

## Family Primulaceae

### COWSLIP
*Primula veris*

A favourite country wild flower which must be protected and tended to ensure that it continues growing and seeding in the areas natural to it. A perennial with oblong, ovate, veined leaves with crinkly surfaces, forming first a rosette and then bearing the nodding umbel-like clusters of orange-yellow flowers in a tubular light green calyx.

**Cultivation and uses:** by seed in autumn or division of root clumps in spring or autumn. Seeds of many wild plants can now be obtained from reputable seed firms. Young leaves and petals can be used in salads, but it is good to let cowslips naturalize somewhere in the garden just for the pleasure of their presence.

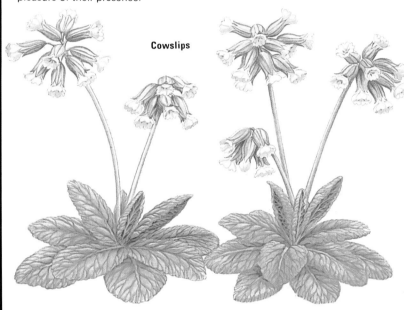

**Cowslips**

### PRIMROSE
*Primula vulgaris*

Well-known perennial spring flower with obovate leaves, deeply veined and wrinkled, and hairy on the underside. The single pale yellow flowers, which grow on a reddish hairy stalk, are tubular at the base and divide into 5 heart-shaped petals.

**Cultivation:** by seed or division of the rootstock. Wild plants should not be dug up (seed can be obtained from almost any seed firm). Hybrids of cowslips, oxlips, primroses and polyanthus will readily occur, and particularly interesting ones can be propagated by division of rootstock to ensure that the progeny comes true.

**Uses:** the tender young leaves and flowers can be used in salads, as they were in the magnificent 'sallets' of Elizabethan times which included 20 or 30 different kinds of leaves, flowers, roots and herbs. The flowers may be candied, using the method described for peppermint leaves, and primrose flower tea is a gentle sedative. An ointment can be made from the plant for treating skin complaints and stiff joints. The primulas are a group of plants which may cause skin eruptions when handled by those unfortunate enough to be allergic to them.

## Family Resedaceae

### MIGNONETTE
*Reseda odorata*

A hardy annual at first forming a rosette of lanceolate leaves and then developing square stems with alternate leaves. The spikes of tiny flowers which bloom in summer have conspicuous orange stamens which almost obscure the white petals. The whole plant has a rather sprawling habit and grows to 12–16in.

**Cultivation:** from seed sown in spring in the place where it is to flower. It will grow in most soils but should not be overcrowded by other plants.

**Uses:** the glorious scent of this rather insignificant-looking herb is the main reason for growing it. The ancient Egyptians cherished it for its perfume and buried wreaths of mignonette with their dead. Its specific name comes from the Latin *resedo*, to appease or soothe, and it was thought to be a sedative and have healing properties. During the 16th century it was a popular pot plant in France, favoured by the Empress Josephine for its scent. The fashion spread to England and in the 19th century it was said that 'all London smelled of Mignonette', as France was said to smell of coffee. In France the plant is grown commercially for its oil which is used in perfumery. Weld (*R. luteola*) grows as an erect spike. It has been an important dye plant since prehistoric times and gives a range of good yellows according to the mordants and materials used.

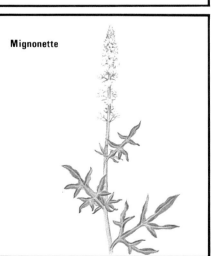

**Mignonette**

# Family Rosaceae

## AGRIMONY
(Church Steeples, Cocklebur)
*Agrimonia eupatoria*
An erect downy perennial with reddish hairy stems (to 32in). It has serrated lanceolate pinnate leaves and leaflets, the undersides greyish with soft hairs. Its slender tapering flower stalks (from which come the common name of Church Steeples) have many deep yellow 5-petalled flowers (2–4in) opening first from the base of the spike, from midsummer. The fruit capsules, at first green then turning to tan colour, have hooked bristles which attach themselves to anything touching them, hence the name Cocklebur.
**Cultivation:** by seed or division of root. Self-seeds freely and will grow on most soils in a sunny position.
**Uses:** at one time a common roadside herb, less plentiful now as verges are often sprayed or cut before plants can seed down. Agrimony was taken as a good spring tonic, as a tea for cystitis and, externally, used to bathe sores and wounds. A natural antibiotic which soothes inflammation, it is an effective sore throat gargle. It was an important ingredient of the famous *eau de arquebusade*, a lotion originally made from herbs to treat those injured by an arquebus or musket. Gerard claims that 'a decoction of the leaves is good for them that have naughty livers'. It is one of those wholesome herbs that may be safely taken for pleasure and will almost certainly be beneficial. Herb teas, or tisanes, are becoming more popular and a tea made from agrimony has a delicate apricot-like flavour. The herb will produce a good yellow dye.

## SALAD BURNET
*Sanguisorba minor (Poterium sanguisorba)*
A short-lived perennial with first a rosette of round to ovate, serrated pinnate leaflets, developing branching reddish stems (to 14in) with leaves arranged alternately. The panicles of flowers are in small round heads of florets, with protruding red-brown stamens for wind pollination.
**Cultivation:** by seed or carefully dividing the root in spring. It will grow in most soils. After flowering the stems should be cut back unless they have already been harvested for drying or are needed to ripen seed. Fresh leaf growth will emerge and survives most winters.
**Uses:** wild burnet, usually browsed by sheep on cliffs or downland, has a refreshing smell of cucumber when trodden on. This flavour, which seems to be combined with that of hazelnuts, makes the tender leaves an attractive addition to salads and imparts a cool flavour to summer drinks, fruit cups and punch. It can be used, fresh or dried, in wine making. It is another styptic herb which will arrest bleeding, and because of its astringency can be taken as an infusion for diarrhoea and to treat piles.

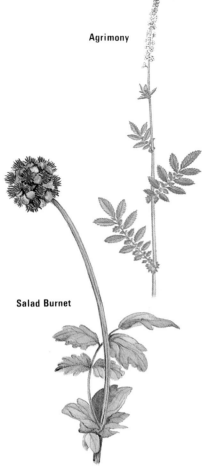

Agrimony

Salad Burnet

Meadowsweet

## MEADOWSWEET
(Queen of the meadow)
*Filipendula ulmaria*
A hardy perennial with a thick rootstock from which reddish stems grow up to 40in. The pinnate, ovate, toothed leaves are downy on the undersides and arranged alternately in two large and two small pairs. The dense corymbs of tiny creamy flowers are sweetly scented from early summer and the leaves are subtly fragrant.
**Cultivation:** from division of root in spring or autumn. A moisture-loving plant, meadowsweet will thrive on heavy soils.
**Uses:** meadowsweet contains salicylic acid from which aspirin (the word comes from *spiraea*) was first derived. Nowadays aspirin is produced synthetically but meadowsweet is still taken as an infusion for rheumatic and arthritic complaints and as a pleasant and gentle sedative. A tea made from flowers of meadowsweet and elder is good to take at the onset of a cold or feverish condition, so it is worth drying the flowers for winter use. The flowers and leaves can be used in salads and soups.

## WILD STRAWBERRY
*Fragaria vesca*
A low-growing hairy perennial on woody rootstock from which runners spread and form new roots. The leaf consists of three pointed, ovate leaflets with serrated edges and a long terminal point. They are strongly veined and shiny on the surface; the undersides paler with hairs. The flowers, borne on upright stems, have 5 broad white petals, and there are small round fragrant fruits.
**Cultivation:** by detaching runners and planting in good compost to encourage strong roots. Varieties of alpine strawberries can be obtained from many nurseries and will spread and naturalize in a position which gets a little shade as well as sun.
**Uses:** the fruits contain vitamin C and are good in fruit salads and summer drinks and give a special flavour to jam made from cultivated strawberries. An infusion of the leaves and flowers makes a refreshing tisane which, when cooled, may be used to bathe the face on hot summer days.

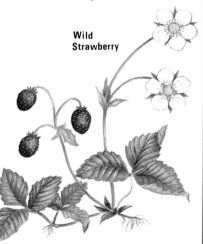

Wild Strawberry

# Family Rubiaceae

## WOODRUFF
(Sweet Woodruffe)
*Asperula odorata*
A low-growing carpeting perennial (to 10in) rooting on angular, erect square stems. The leaves are in whorls of 6–8 lanceolate leaflets, terminating in loose clusters of tubular, white, 4-lobed flowers.
**Cultivation:** by division of the slender-rooted stems in spring or autumn. It will grow best in semi-shade in a humus-rich soil and provides an attractive ground cover.
**Uses:** when the leaves are dried they have a delicious new-mown hay scent which comes from the coumarin released from the plant. The herb is excellent as a tisane, or used in summer fruit drinks and white wine. It has a carminative action and will help to settle an upset stomach. It makes a welcome addition to pot pourri and on its own in open bowls will give an elusive fragrance to a room.

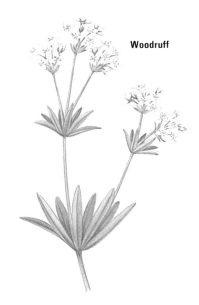

Woodruff

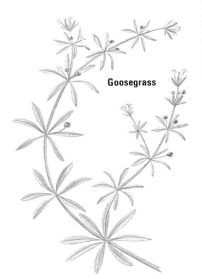

Goosegrass

## GOOSEGRASS
(Cleavers, Everlasting Friendship)
*Galium aparine*
An annual which appears very early in the year and spreads rapidly. The squared stems and leaves are all furnished with hooked bristles which assist it to climb into hedges and through nearby vegetation to a length of over 40in. Groups of linear leaves and stipules are arranged in whorls at the nodes of the angular stems and tiny whitish flowers are borne on stalks springing from the axils of the leaves, ripening to round seed vessels also covered with hooked bristles. The plant 'cleaves' or clings to anything it touches including any other plant material, animal, fur, wool, or clothing of passers by, thus dispersing itself over a wide area.
**Cultivation and uses:** from seed sown in autumn when ripe, but should only be grown in a wild part of the garden. The young plant is edible; although bitter to taste, it may be chopped and eaten raw or cooked as a green vegetable. From late summer the ripe seeds can be stripped off in handfuls, roasted and ground as an alternative to coffee (the coffee shrub *Coffea arabica* from which the coffee berries of commerce are gathered, belongs to the same natural order as goosegrass). Used as a lotion, it is considered an effective treatment for skin eruptions and taken internally as a tea can help to soothe inflammations of the bladder.

# Family Rutaceae

## RUE
(Herb of grace)
*Ruta graveolens*
A bushy perennial with woody stems and alternate blue-green leaves with deeply divided leaflets. The yellow flowers have 4 separated petals and prominent stamens. The cultivar, Jackman's Blue rue, has denser spatulate foliage of deep blue-green.
**Cultivation:** by seed or cuttings in spring. Jackman's Blue rue is best propagated from cuttings to ensure that it comes true. Well-drained soil and a position where the plants get some shade in the heat of the day seems to suit them best.
**Uses:** for hundreds of years this herb was used in the treatment of disease and bunches were carried to give protection from pestilence. It was an ingredient of the Vinegar of the Four Thieves (see garlic) and of an infamous medication known as Gilbert's Puppy Dog Ointment concocted by an Englishman, Gilbertus Anglicus, in the 15th century: 'Take a very fat puppy dog and skin him; then take the juice of cucumber, rue and pellitory; berries of ivy and juniper; fat of vulture, fox, goose and bear in equal parts; stuff the puppy therewith and boil him; add wax to the grease that floats on the surface and make therefrom an ointment.' Rue also had pleasanter uses. Rue water was sprinkled to rid houses of fleas and the sprigs of the herb were used to sprinkle holy water before Mass, hence Shakespeare's reference in 'Hamlet' to the 'herb of grace o' Sundays'. Rue has a strange smell which, with better acquaintance, becomes intriguing rather than unpleasant. A leaf or so may be added to salads and a weak infusion can be drunk as a digestive, but the beauty of its foliage alone is sufficient reason to grow rue. It is said that sage and rue will not flourish if planted near each other, but long experience of growing them in close proximity has not confirmed this. However, as there seems to be an affinity between some plants, there may also be an intolerance. Rue, like primulas and chrysanthemums, can cause skin troubles in those with an allergy to it.

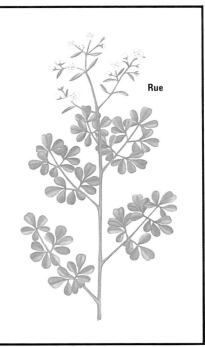

Rue

## Family Scrophulariaceae

**Eyebright**

**Great Mullein**

### EYEBRIGHT
(Euphrasy)
*Euphrasia rostkoviana (E. officinalis)*
A small erect branching annual (to 12in) with ovate, sharply-serrated leaves in opposite pairs. The inflorescence comprises short spikes of pale mauve-white flowers with two purple-veined lips, the larger lower one with three cleft lobes and a yellow spot at the throat. There are glandular hairs on the calyx. Eyebright, which grows wild on downs and heaths, is semi-parasitic on some species of grass so is not easy to establish in cultivation.

**Uses:** the markings of the flower may once have suggested bloodshot eyes and its main use in herbal medicine is still in opthalmic treatments. Milton brings the use of eyebright into his poetry, giving it early fame by writing of the Archangel Michael removing the film from Adam's eyes with euphrasia and rue after his fall from grace in the garden of Eden 'for he had much to see'. In many parts of the world it is regarded as a specific cure for inflammation of the eyes. Owing to the problem of cultivating it as one would other herbs in the garden, cooled and carefully-strained infusions of loose-strife, fennel or comfrey can be substituted to bathe sore eyes.

### GREAT MULLEIN
(Beggar's Blanket)
*Verbascum thapsus*
A stout biennial (to 40–52in). From the taproot in the first year grows a flat rosette of downy flannel-like leaves (12in or more in length), entire, ovate-lanceolate. In the second year the leaves diminish in size as they ascend the stems. The stems, sometimes branching, terminate in dense spikes of yellow flowers with 5 flattened petal-like lobes joined at the base of the corolla which are out of character with the two-lipped flowers of this family.

**Cultivation:** by seed sown in autumn or spring. It will grow in most reasonably well-drained soils and is usually found growing wild on waste ground and dry hedge banks.

**Uses:** great mullein has over thirty common names (candlewick plant, hag's taper, feltwort and many more) all suggesting uses to which this herb has been put. The names beggar's blanket and old man's flannel suggest the warmth the large downy leaves would give to chilly bones when tucked inside thin garments. Feltwort describes the felt-like texture of the leaves. Their woolly surface used to be rolled off and used as a wick for lights, while the whole spike was dipped in tallow and carried as a torch. The flowers are used as an infusion or made into a syrup with honey for all chest complaints. When dried, the leaves and flowers can be combined with herbs like coltsfoot and clover to make a herbal smoking mixture for bronchial troubles. The emollient properties of the herb can be made use of in poultices and fomentations, and a yellow dye is made from the flowers.

## Family Tropaeolaceae

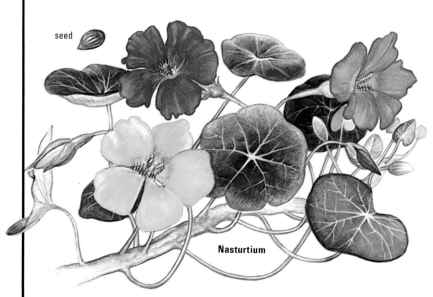

seed

**Nasturtium**

### NASTURTIUM
*Tropaeolum majus*
An annual herb with entire round leaves (2–4in), a little wavy at the edges, growing on brittle pale green leaf stalks. The spurred flowers (2–3in) vary in colour from pale yellow to bronze and shades of red.

**Cultivation:** the large seeds are sown in spring spaced 4–8in apart and pushed 1¼in into the soil. Nasturtium thrives happily in a sunny place but will give a welcome patch of colour in semi-shade.

**Uses:** in addition to its ornamental interest as a bush plant, trailer or climber it is a salad herb which may be used in place of watercress *(Nasturtium officinale)*. It gets its name from the hot cress flavour which has a tendency to act as a 'nasturtium' or nose twister! The green unripe seeds can be soaked in salted water for 12 hours, rinsed in fresh water and then packed into bottles with spiced or dill vinegar poured over them. They are used instead of capers, but will taste better if kept for 6 months first. The leaves contain vitamin C and have a natural antibiotic action.

# Family Umbelliferae

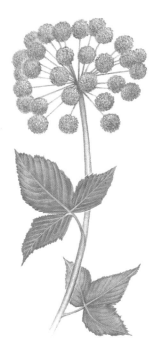

**Angelica**

## ANGELICA
*Angelica Archangelica*
Although botanically classified as a biennial this herb may live for several years. On thick branching roots it makes substantial growth the first year into a clump of hollow stems with light green leaves, subdivided into leaflets with serrated edges. In the second year the central flower stem grows up to 40–60in, carrying rounded umbels of tiny yellow-green florets, followed by masses of flattened oval seeds.
**Cultivation:** the viable life of angelica seed is short and they should be sown in autumn when fully ripe and not kept until spring. The young seedlings will lose their leaves for the winter (as the parent plant also dies down) but they reappear in spring, usually in large quantities. This big plant needs adequate moisture in the soil to maintain its growth and does well in a heavy soil. Angelica flourishes in Lapland and the Scandinavian countries so there is little doubt about its hardiness for garden cultivation. In the past it was regarded as an important medicinal herb; legend tells that it acquired the distinctive title of Archangelica because the Archangel Michael appeared in a dream to a monk in time of plague, instructing the people to chew angelica root as a protective measure. It is used in the treatment of bronchitis and to stimulate appetite in those debilitated by illness. A pleasant after-dinner tisane made from the leaves acts as a carminative. The stalks

give interesting results when blended with rhubarb, gooseberry or marrow for jams and conserves, or when making elderflower wine. It is an ingredient of vermouth, Benedictine and other liqueurs. The candied stalks are familiar as cake and dessert decoration. Home-candied angelica is delicious and, although the process is spread over a couple of days, it is very simple to make. Using only the tender basal stalks towards the end of May, cut them into 4in lengths, put in a pan with just enough water to cover them and boil gently until soft. Drain and strip off the fine outer skin. Weigh the stalks and add the same amount of sugar and leave in a covered bowl (not metal) for two days. They will have made syrup by this time and should be brought to the boil and simmered gently until the angelica clears. A drop of good green colouring may be added if liked. Drain through a colander, dip the sticks in icing sugar and put on a cake rack in a cool oven to dry off; but do not allow them to get too hard. Store between several layers of greaseproof paper in airtight boxes.

## ANISE
*Pimpinella anisum*
A tender half-hardy annual (to 20in) with a thin taproot and erect stems bearing broad, deeply-lobed and toothed leaves at the base and finely cut narrow leaflets up the stem. Branching flower stems terminate in compound umbels of tiny white or cream flowers, followed by ribbed seeds, brown when ripe.
**Cultivation:** by seed sown in early summer outside or a little earlier in pots indoors for protection if the weather is poor.
**Uses:** the warm aromatic flavour of aniseed is familiar to most people. An excellent digestive, the seeds can be chewed after a meal or a tisane made from seeds or leaves. It can be used instead of fennel to dress fish, with egg dishes and in salads.

**Anise**

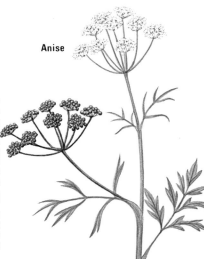

**Caraway**

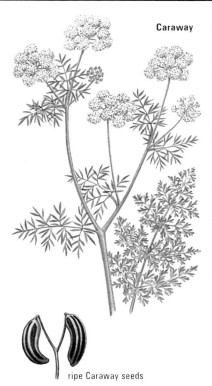

ripe Caraway seeds

## CARAWAY
*Carum carvi*
A biennial with a slender taproot and erect stems (to 20in), the leaves consisting of many finely cut leaflets. The flowers are in compound umbels of tiny white florets followed by narrow ridged green seeds ($\frac{1}{4}$in) which are brown when ripe.
**Cultivation:** from seed sown in early autumn the young plants overwinter and come into flower late the following spring, ripening seed in early summer. The plant dies after seeding but on light soil will self-sow and continue the cycle. A light well-drained soil and sunny position is advised.
**Uses:** for 5000 years or so this herb has acted as a carminative and cured digestive troubles in children and adults. It is the flavouring agent of the liqueur Kummel and is used in cheeses, cakes, breads, biscuits, with fruit dishes and vegetables. Those who dislike the grittiness of caraway seeds in cakes and buns may like to try using the seeds when they are green and succulent, at which time they impart their flavour but are not hard. The roots, grated raw in salads or cooked like small parsnips as a vegetable, are good served with pork. The leaves can be used for salads and soups. In the past caraway was recommended for 'pale faced girls', perhaps because it stimulated their appetites and so made them look rosier, and it was put into love potions to encourage faithfulness.

## CHERVIL
*Anthriscus cerefolium*

An attractive fragrant biennial (to 12in) with deeply cut ferny leaves consisting of pinnate and terminal leaflets. It has umbels of tiny white flowers and thin seeds ($\frac{1}{4}$–$\frac{1}{2}$in).

**Cultivation:** seed is best sown in late summer when it ripens on the plant; the young seedlings will overwinter and grow on in spring. If it is to be dried it should be cut as soon as it is big enough to prevent it flowering and seeding; dry weather accelerates this maturing process. The leaves are sometimes tinged with pink, but for drying only the green ones are taken.

**Uses:** this pretty plant with lacy foliage is ornamental to grow and the slightly accented anise-flavoured leaves are delicious in salads, with fish, egg and cheese dishes, in sauces, savoury dips and as a garnish on soups. Its flavour is lost in long cooking so it should be used fresh and added at the last moment. It freezes well and makes an interesting alternative to parsley.

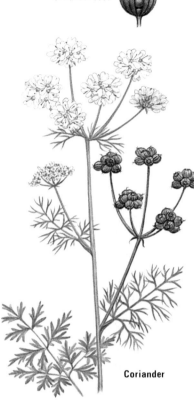

Coriander seed

Coriander

Chervil

## CORIANDER
*Coriandrum sativum*

An annual (20–24in) with erect, branching stems, deeply cut broadly segmented lower leaves and finely feathery upper stem leaves. The pale pink flowers are in light umbels and mature as small round ridged green fruits, biscuit-coloured when ripe.

**Cultivation:** by seed sown as soon as the soil is workable in spring. Covering them with a cloche in their early stages will be helpful. Coriander is fairly hardy and will grow on most soils that are in good condition, but a sunny situation is needed to ripen the seeds.

**Uses:** the flavour of home-grown coriander is superb and it improves as the seeds are stored, which must be when totally dry and in airtight containers. Coriander is an ancient herb widely used in cooking. It is a basic flavouring for curries and is used in chutneys and pickles, with yoghourts and dips, fruit and vegetables. If fresh leaves are wanted, some plants should be discouraged from flowering by cutting out the potential flower stalks to stimulate more leaf growth. The leaves are used in curries and chutneys to serve with curry.

## CUMIN
*Cuminum cyminum*

An annual with a thin taproot, branching slender stems (6–8in) and fine thread-like foliage. The irregular umbels of small pinkish-white flowers mature to ridged seeds similar to those of caraway.

**Cultivation:** sow seed indoors in pots or boxes in spring. In late May or June if the weather is suitable, carefully transplant to a warm, sheltered place. Keep a ball of compost around the plants so as not to disturb the roots.

**Uses:** this is another herb which has been in use for thousands of years as a carminative. The seeds give a warm pungency to curries and stews and are used with courgettes and marrows, in herb vinegars and as a tisane to aid digestion after meals.

## DILL
*Anethum graveolens*

A hardy annual (to 36in) with hollow erect stems and feathery leaves which have finely cut thread-like leaflets of a bluish-green. The inflorescense is a dainty rounded compound umbel of many clusters of tiny yellow florets.

**Cultivation:** from seed sown in spring where it is to grow because, like most of the other annual umbellifers, it does not transplant well. It will grow in most soils but likes a sunny site.

**Uses:** though similar in appearance dill and fennel have quite different scents and flavours and if the liquorice taste of fennel is not liked, dill may be found pleasant as an alternative. It is a popular herb in Scandinavian countries, the Norse word *dilla* means to lull. Dill water, a simple infusion of the leaves or seeds, is used to soothe babies with wind or stomach upsets. Use freshly chopped with new potatoes, peas, fish, omelettes, salads and pickles.

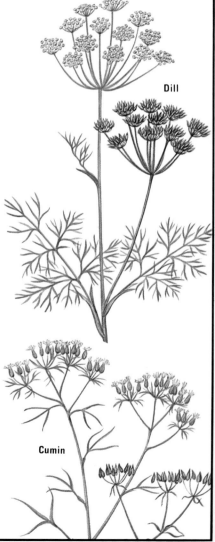

Dill

Cumin

## FENNEL
*Foeniculum vulgare (F. officinalis)*
A tall hardy perennial with a thick tap-root and hollow stems (40–60in). The feathery leaves are formed of bright green thread-like leaflets. The flower is a flat umbel of tiny yellow florets.
**Cultivation:** by seed sown in spring or autumn. This herb will grow in most soils in an open situation and self-sows freely on light soils.
**Uses:** in spring the tender young stalks can be peeled of their outer skin (like rhubarb) and eaten raw like celery or used in salads. Sprays of fennel leaves cooked with fish are best removed before serving and fresh ones used as a garnish, or in a sauce served with the dish. Fennel is 'a gallant expeller of the wind' and at one time was thought to be a slimming herb, possibly because eating it is alleged to take away the pangs of hunger. It is also said to be most soothing when used to bathe sore eyes. Sweet or Florence fennel (*F. dulce*) is the annual variety. Its swollen stem bases can be freshly cut and eaten raw as a salad herb or cooked and served with oil, butter or a sauce.

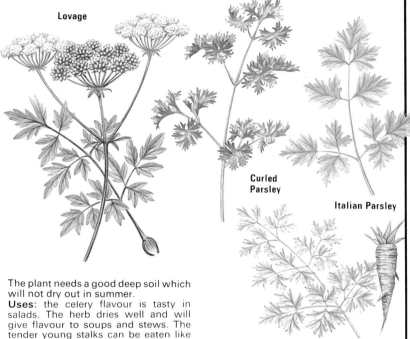

Lovage

Curled Parsley

Italian Parsley

Hamburg Parsley

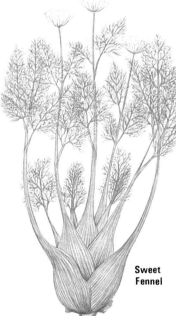

Sweet Fennel

## LOVAGE
*Levisticum officinale*
A hairless perennial dying down in winter. From the fleshy rootstock grow stout hollow ridged stems (to 60in) when the plant is mature. The yellowish-green leaves consist of 3 serrated ovate or deeply indented leaflets and the small yellow flowers which appear in late summer are in terminal compound umbels.
**Cultivation:** from seed in early autumn or late spring. The roots can be cut to give a piece of root with a bud or 'eye' attached and replanted in spring.

The plant needs a good deep soil which will not dry out in summer.
**Uses:** the celery flavour is tasty in salads. The herb dries well and will give flavour to soups and stews. The tender young stalks can be eaten like sticks of celery. Lovage aids digestion, acts as a mild diuretic and may be helpful to sufferers from rheumatism.

## PARSLEY
(Moss curled parsley)
*Petroselinum crispum*
A biennial on a short taproot with deeply divided leaflets which form the familiar curly rich green foliage. If allowed to flower the ridged stalks produce umbels of pale yellowish-green tiny florets.
**Cultivation and uses:** sow seed in late summer or spring. Parsley needs a good moisture-retaining soil and will do well in partial shade as well as full sunlight. The flower stalks should be removed to prolong leaf production. Italian parsley *(P. hortense filicinum)* has flat deeply indented trifoliate leaves and a strong flavour, and Hamburg Parsley *(P. sativum tuberosum)* which grows like a parsnip or sometimes like a turnip, may be grated raw for salads or cooked as a vegetable. All are grown from seed. Parsley, familiar as a garnish and flavouring for stuffings, soups and sauces, stimulates the appetite and acts as a diuretic. Eaten after garlic, it helps to destroy the odour.

## SWEET CICELY
*Myrrhis odorata*
A hardy perennial dying down in winter. From the large rootstock buds develop into hollow, branching stems (to 38in) with bright green hairy, deeply segmented pinnate leaflets, some with white blotches. The tiny white flowers are in compound umbels (2–4in across).
**Cultivation:** by division of root crown or seed sown in late autumn and left to stratify in the cold soil of winter and germinate in spring. The plant likes a moisture-retaining soil.
**Uses:** all parts of the plant are anise-flavoured and sweet to taste. The young stems can be peeled and eaten. Leaves and stems added to early gooseberries, rhubarb or later to plums which may not be fully ripe, will take away the tartness of the fruit and less sugar can be used in cooking them. Sweet cicely is used by diabetics as a sugar substitute.

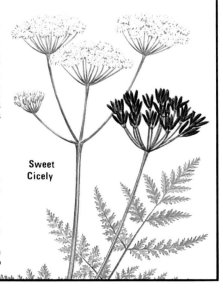

Sweet Cicely

## Family Urticaceae

### NETTLE
*Urtica dioica*

A persistent perennial growing over 40in in height from creeping rootstock, with erect stems bearing opposite and alternate pairs of sharply serrated heart-shaped leaves which are hairy and stinging. Male and female flowers are on different plants and the infloresence, coming from the axils of the leaves, hangs as drooping racemes of small greenish florets without petals, which are wind pollinated.

**Cultivation and uses:** any pieces of rhizome pulled off and replanted will quickly establish. Nettle is not a herb usually encouraged in cultivation – the effort is rather to eradicate it – but in a wild area there are reasons for letting it flourish. Probably one of the most underestimated growing herbs, it is an invaluable plant which has been a source of food, medicine, fibre and dyes since the Bronze Age. Among its known constituents are iron, calcium, potassium and other trace elements, vitamins A and C, and histamine. It has a wide application for treating internal and external bleeding, haemorrhoids, and many skin complaints, including eczema and urticaria (nettle rash). It can lower the blood sugar level and is used in the treatment of rheumatism. In the past it was a vital spring green vegetable, helping to purify blood and clear up vitamin deficiency ailments caused by poor winter diet; while nettle tea and nettle beer were favourite spring beverages. It is richer in iron and vitamins than spinach. Cook the young leaves in the water adhering to them after they have been washed, add a little olive oil or butter, and serve with poached eggs, grated cheese, nutmeg or a squeeze of lemon juice. Combine them with leeks or watercress for soup. The plants contain natural sugar, starch and protein. When the plants are allowed to grow they become coarse and are not suitable for eating, but if cut down to ground level tender young leaves will soon come again. The mature plants were once used as an important fibre in clothmaking. It was an alternative to cotton and in some cases considered superior to flax. Nettles have also been employed in the manufacture of paper, of commercial chlorophyll, and as a dye. Cut, dried nettle is fed to poultry, goats and cattle; and the caterpillars of many butterflies – comma, small tortoiseshell, red admiral, peacock and painted lady – feed on the leaves. An infusion of nettles can be used as a feed for houseplants.

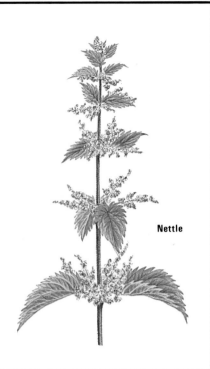

Nettle

## Family Valerianaceae

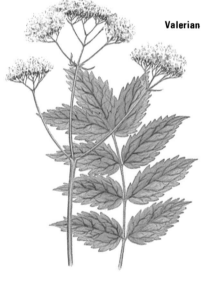

Valerian

### VALERIAN
(Phu)
*Valeriana officinalis*

A hardy perennial with slender rhizomes radiating from the centre of the rootstock. In spring lanceolate, pinnate radical leaves, some toothed, form a basal clump from which grow the ridged, hollow, flowering stems (36–48in) with terminal corymbs of pale pink tubular florets.

**Cultivation:** division of rootstock is easily achieved by detaching plantlets from the outside of the parent plant. Valerian is found wild in ditches and moist places and will do best in soil that is moisture-retaining and rich in humus.

**Uses:** one of the oldest-known nervine herbs, it is used as a sedative and anti-spasmodic in the treatment of nervous and anxiety problems. The root is dried and in the process emits a powerful tom-cat smell, hence its ancient name of 'phu'. The time of year at which the root is dug affects its potency.

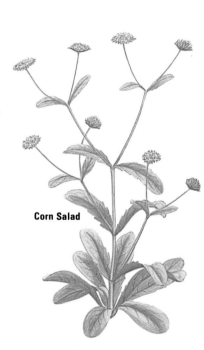

Corn Salad

### CORN SALAD
(Lamb's Lettuce, Loblollie)
*Valerianella locusta (V. olitoria)*

A hardy annual with opposite oblong leaves on much-branched stems (to 12in). Terminal clusters of tiny pale lilac florets are found sparsely in the axils of the leaves.

**Cultivation:** by seed sown in succession from spring. Late summer sowing will give plants which grow on into the winter. Corn salad likes most soils and an open situation. It self-sows freely.

**Uses:** an easily grown salad herb of the cut-and-come-again type, best used when the leaves are young. It is hardy for winter use and was popular in the days when vegetables were scarce as a good tonic and blood cleansing food.

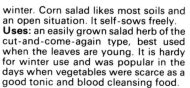

## Family Verbenaceae

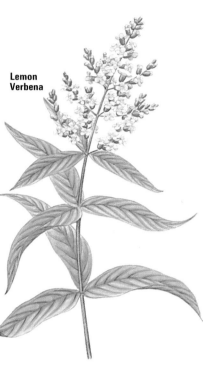

Lemon
Verbena

### VERBENA, LEMON
*Aloysia triphylla (Lippia citriodora)*
A deciduous shrub (to 40in) with branching stems, lemon-scented, lanceolate leaves and slender flower spikes with pale lavender two-lipped flowers.
**Cultivation:** by cuttings in late spring. Verbena should be protected in winter unless growing in temperate sheltered conditions. It looks very dead with dry pale leafless branches in winter, but in spring buds will break from the nodes.
**Uses:** delicious as a tea, to garnish melon and other fruits and to flavour sponge cakes. When dried, it can be put in bowls to give fragrance to a room and used as an ingredient of pot pourri.

### VERVAIN
*Verbena officinalis*
A perennial herb with fibrous roots and a bushy growth of hairless, angular branching stems (28–36in). The basal leaves are broad ovate, deeply indented and toothed; the stem leaves lanceolate, in opposite pairs. The two-lipped lavender-coloured flowers open from the base of a slender pointed spike.
**Cultivation:** from seed or division of root. This herb likes a fairly dry, sunny position and although the flowers are displayed sparsely on the spikes, their effect is dainty and elegant over many weeks in summer.
**Uses:** the history of vervain is confused. A herb of priests, druids and witches, it was regarded with fear in case it was used in harmful witchcraft, and with respect in the hope that it might give protection from the evil eye. It is still used as a sedative for nervous complaints and as a general tonic. It has proved beneficial in the treatment of certain skin troubles which may have been caused by nervous tension.

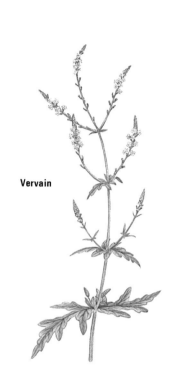

Vervain

## Family Violaceae

### VIOLET
*Viola odorata*
A hardy perennial (to 8in). The fibrous creeping roots spread by stolons rooting at the nodes and making new plants which, by repeating the process, soon cover the area around the original plant. The dark green heart-shaped leaves with crenate edges grow on long stalks and emit an elusive violet perfume before the flowers open. The self-fertile flowers are carried on long stems which curve over at their tips to carry a single bloom. These are commonly violet-blue but many shades exist and some flowers are double.
**Cultivation:** from seed or detached rooted stolons set in a humus-rich soil in a position with some shade. Because the plant propagates itself so freely it soon exhausts the ground on which it is growing and generous dressings of leafmould must be put down to prevent the soil from drying out. A violet bed benefits from being cleared of all the

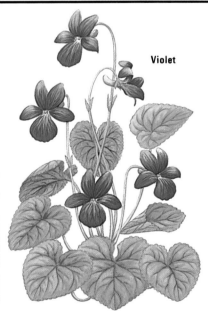

Violet

old plants every couple of years.
**Uses:** the scent and beauty of the violet have been praised by poets and writers since early classical times and there can be few people who would feel anything but pleasure in being the recipient of a bunch of violets at anytime of the year. The commercial production of violets is an important part of the flower-producing industry, and in Europe they are still grown to a limited extent for the production of violet perfume which, like lavender, remains constantly popular. The flowers were made into syrups, wines and cosmetic washes; eaten in salads, fried in oil and candied; and used medicinally for skin complaints and as poultices for ulcers.

# GLOSSARY

**achene:** a small nut-like fruit; a carpel containing a single seed.

**annual:** plant that lives for one year only.

**antispasmodic:** relieves convulsive or spasmodic pains.

**antiviral:** a substance capable of attacking some virus infections.

**axil:** the angle between the stem and the upper side of the leaf stalk.

**biennial:** plant that is sown in one year to flower and die the next.

**bract:** modified leaf-like structure.

**bulbil:** small or immature bulb.

**calyx:** collective word for total number of sepals.

**capsule:** vessel containing seeds which when ripe usually splits open and expels the seeds at random.

**carminative:** a substance which relieves flatulence.

**carpel:** a division in the seed vessel.

**clone:** a product of vegetable propagation, being identical in all characteristics to that of the parent.

**compound umbel:** umbel, itself made up of umbels.

**cordate:** heart-shaped.

**corm:** bulb-like underground stem.

**corolla:** collective word for total number of petals.

**corymb:** a raceme where lower flower-stalks are proportionally larger.

**cultivar:** a variety or form taken from the wild and cultivated as a clone.

**cyme:** flower cluster in which each growing point ends in a flower, the oldest flowers being at the top or centre of the cluster.

**deciduous:** a plant that loses its leaves in winter.

**disc florets:** small tubular florets typical of the Compositae family, forming tightly-packed yellow centre of flower (e.g. yarrow or daisy).

**diuretic:** a substance which stimulates the flow of urine.

**drill:** a shallow indentation or trench in which to sow seeds or lay rhizomes.

**elliptic:** oval with narrowed ends.

**emollient:** a substance which softens skin.

**febrifuge:** a medicinal substance to reduce fevers.

**fibrous roots:** many slender massed roots of fibrous nature (e.g. basil, chives).

**florets:** small individual flowers making up a head or cluster.

**hastate:** arrow-shaped.

**'heel':** the heel-shaped base of a cutting when a shoot is pulled downwards to detach it from a stem for propagation.

**histamine:** a substance present in the body which when released into the blood protects against infection from burns or wounds.

**inflorescence:** the arrangement or grouping of flowers on a plant.

**island bed:** a bed situated on a lawn or area to be viewed from all sides. It is best to put tall plants in the centre and graduate heights down to low growing plants at the front edges.

**internode:** the space between nodes on a stem.

**lanceolate:** narrow with tapering ends.

**linear:** strap-shaped.

**mucilage:** a gummy, glutinous substance found in some plants, often soothing to inflamed areas of skin.

**mulch:** rotted leaves, lawn mowings, peat, compost and shredded bark used to spread over the ground around plants to give protection and help to conserve moisture in the soil. Mulch should not be spread on dry soil as it prevents the rain soaking down to the roots for some time.

**node:** the 'joint' on a stem from which leaf, flower or other stem buds develop.

**ovate:** egg-shaped in outline.

**panicle:** a raceme with branching stalks.

**pappus:** fine hairy down which acts as a parachute for the dispersal of airborne seeds (e.g. dandelion and hemp agrimony).

**perennial:** plant that lives for several years.

**pinnate:** arrangement of leaflets in opposite pairs on common stalks.

**raceme:** cylindrical head of stalked flowers.

**radical leaves:** those growing directly from the crown of the root (e.g. elecampane).

**ray florets:** small flowers having elongated or strap-shaped lobes, as the outer white florets of yarrow or daisy flowers.

**reniform:** kidney-shaped.

**rhizomes:** an underground stem that produces roots and leafy shoots.

**rootstocks:** gardener's term for the two or three year old mature roots which may be divided up, or from which growing buds can be cut, to form new young plants.

**sepal:** usually, green, leaf-like part of flower in ring beneath petals, enclosing flower in bud.

**spike:** cylindrical head of unstalked flowers.

**'sport':** a term used to describe a shoot or part of a plant which is out of character with the usual form and only by vegetative propagation can maintain its individual nature.

**stamen:** male part of flower made up of pollen-producing anther on stalk.

**stigma:** tip of female part of flower which receives the pollen.

**stipules:** pairs of small, modified leaf-like structures at the base of the leaf stalk, giving protection to the bud.

**stolon:** a horizontal stem at soil level which produces a new plant at its tip.

**strobile:** a cone shaped inflorescence made up of overlapping scales (e.g. hop).

**style:** stalk of stigma leading to ovary.

**styptic:** an astringent substance used to arrest bleeding.

**taproot:** a thick, often tapering root, usually storing food (e.g. carrot, Hamburg parsley).

**tisane:** an infusion of dried herbs.

**umbel:** umbrella-shaped flower-head in which equal flower-stalks arise from same point on stem.

**umbellifer:** plant in the Carrot family.

**viable:** capable of producing living growth; that is, germination of seeds.

**vulnerary:** a substance used in the treatment or healing of wounds.

**whorl:** leaves or flowers arranged around stem in a ring.

In this book, the herbs are grouped alphabetically in botanical families, the common name first, then the genus and species in Latin. If we take Peppermint as an example: the family is Labiateae (with lipped flowers), the genus is *Mentha* (mint) and the species *piperita* (with a peppery, hot taste). Common names vary from one place to another but Latin names are adopted internationally, so a knowledge of the latter makes identification of plants easier and more positive. The glossary below explains some of the Latin words used to describe species:

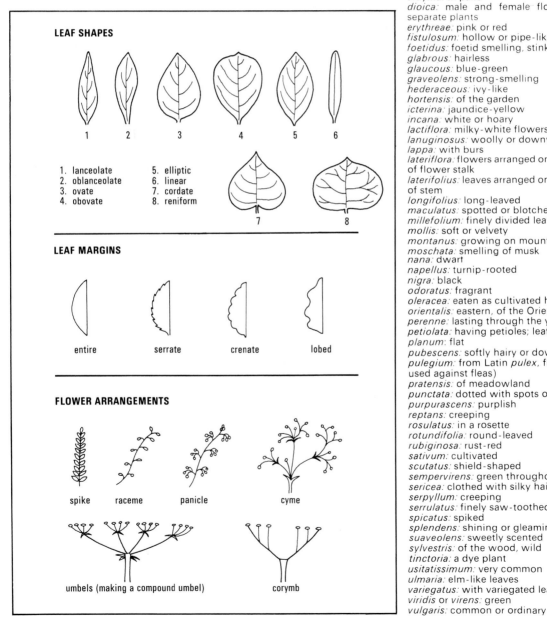

**LEAF SHAPES**

1  2  3  4  5  6

1. lanceolate
2. oblanceolate
3. ovate
4. obovate
5. elliptic
6. linear
7. cordate
8. reniform

7  8

**LEAF MARGINS**

entire    serrate    crenate    lobed

**FLOWER ARRANGEMENTS**

spike    raceme    panicle    cyme

umbels (making a compound umbel)    corymb

*acetosa*: acid
*alba*: white
*angustifolia*: narrow-leaved
*aquatica*: growing in or near water
*aureus*: golden
*balsamita*: balsam-scented
*chenopodium*: leaves of goose-foot shape
*citriodorus*: lemon-scented
*crispum*: curled
*didyma*: in pairs
*dioica*: male and female flowers on separate plants
*erythreae*: pink or red
*fistulosum*: hollow or pipe-like stems
*foetidus*: foetid smelling, stinking
*glabrous*: hairless
*glaucous*: blue-green
*graveolens*: strong-smelling
*hederaceous*: ivy-like
*hortensis*: of the garden
*icterina*: jaundice-yellow
*incana*: white or hoary
*lactiflora*: milky-white flowers
*lanuginosus*: woolly or downy
*lappa*: with burs
*lateriflora*: flowers arranged on one side of flower stalk
*laterifolius*: leaves arranged on one side of stem
*longifolius*: long-leaved
*maculatus*: spotted or blotched
*millefolium*: finely divided leaves
*mollis*: soft or velvety
*montanus*: growing on mountains
*moschata*: smelling of musk
*nana*: dwarf
*napellus*: turnip-rooted
*nigra*: black
*odoratus*: fragrant
*oleracea*: eaten as cultivated herb
*orientalis*: eastern, of the Orient
*perenne*: lasting through the year
*petiolata*: having petioles; leaf stalks
*planum*: flat
*pubescens*: softly hairy or downy
*pulegium*: from Latin *pulex*, flea (to be used against fleas)
*pratensis*: of meadowland
*punctata*: dotted with spots or glands
*purpurascens*: purplish
*reptans*: creeping
*rosulatus*: in a rosette
*rotundifolia*: round-leaved
*rubiginosa*: rust-red
*sativum*: cultivated
*scutatus*: shield-shaped
*sempervirens*: green throughout year
*sericea*: clothed with silky hairs
*serpyllum*: creeping
*serrulatus*: finely saw-toothed
*spicatus*: spiked
*splendens*: shining or gleaming
*suaveolens*: sweetly scented
*sylvestris*: of the wood, wild
*tinctoria*: a dye plant
*usitatissimum*: very common
*ulmaria*: elm-like leaves
*variegatus*: with variegated leaves
*viridis* or *virens*: green
*vulgaris*: common or ordinary

# INDEX